Monthly Nutrition Companion
31 Days to a Healthier Lifestyle

Written for The American Dietetic Association by
Roberta Larson Duyff, MS, RD, CFCS
Duyff Associates
St. Louis, Missouri

The American Dietetic Association Reviewers:
Sharon C. Denny, MS, RD
National Center for Nutrition
 and Dietetics
Chicago, Illinois

Mindy Hermann, MBA, RD
The Hermann Group
Mt. Kisko, New York

Lisa Stollman, MA, RD
Preventive Nutrition Services
Northport, New York

Technical Editor:
Betsy Hornick, MS, RD
The American Dietetic Association
Chicago, Illinois

JOHN WILEY & SONS, INC.
New York • Chichester • Weinheim • Brisbane • Singapore • Toronto

THE AMERICAN DIETETIC ASSOCIATION is the largest group of food and nutrition professionals in the world. As the advocate of the profession, the ADA serves the public by promoting optimal nutrition, health, and well-being.

To learn more about nutrition or obtain a referral to an RD in your area, call the ADA/National Center for Nutrition and Dietetics Hot Line at (800) 366-1655. Visit ADA on the World Wide Web at http://www.eatright.org.

This book is printed on acid-free paper. ⊖

Copyright © 1997 by the American Dietetic Association. All rights reserved

Published by John Wiley & Sons, Inc.
Published simultaneously in Canada
Previously published by Chronimed Publishing

Illustrations by Neverne Covington

The information contained in this book is not intended to serve as a replacement for professional medical advice. Any use of the information in this book is at the reader's discretion. The author and the publisher specifically disclaim any and all liability arising directly or indirectly from the use or application of any information contained in this book. A health care professional should be consulted regarding your specific situation.

ISBN 0-471-34688-8

Printed in the United States of America

10 9 8 7 6 5 4 3 2

Table of Contents

Chapter 1: **Personally Yours** 1
Fit for Change

Chapter 2: **All About You**. 3
Rate Your Plate
Get in Touch
Check Your Weight
Figure Your Waist-to-Hip Ratio
Rate Your "Gait"
Consider Change

Chapter 3: **Eating for Fitness!** 11
Pyramid Your Way to Healthful Eating
Your Foods—Where Do They Fit?
Sizing It All Up
Fluid Assets

Chapter 4: **Making Your Best Moves**. 29
Get Moving: For Health-Smart Reasons!
How to Get Moving

Chapter 5: **Charting Your Course** 33
Build Your Pyramid for Fitness
Get Smart, Get Set, Get Moving!
Stepping to Fitness: Your Personal Goals and Action Plans

Chapter 6: **Your Day-by-Day Companion** 39

When You Need to Know More 181

About Some Nutrients in Food

Sorting the Fat, Saturated Fat, and Cholesterol, Too

Vitamin A: Good Picks

Vitamin C: Not Just From Citrus!

Calcium: How Much in Food?

Iron... From Many Sources

Food's Fiber Factor

Sodium: In Which Foods?

Healthy Weight—For You!

In the Mood for Food!

How to Get Sound Advice About Healthful Eating

Index 201

Chapter One

Personally Yours

WHATEVER YOUR PERSONAL HEALTH GOALS, the *Monthly Nutrition Companion* can help you apply nutrition basics to your lifestyle—one step at a time. Healthful eating and an active lifestyle are both fundamental to your overall health and well-being. In fact, wise food choices and physical activity are partners in promoting fitness.

What does it mean to be fit? Being fit is more than just being free of disease or physically fit. Think of fitness as your optimal good health: physical, emotional, and mental. Being fit gives you a better chance for a higher quality of life, more stamina, a positive outlook—perhaps a longer life, too.

Keeping fit also reduces your risk for many of today's health problems. Heart disease, cancer, and diabetes, for example, are related to food choices and personal lifestyles. Although not addressed in this book, heredity and other lifestyle choices—for example, adequate rest, stress management, not smoking, regular medical checkups, adequate health care, among others—promote your overall health, too. Consider the whole picture as you step toward fitness.

Decisions you can control *over a lifetime* can promote your health—and quality of life. The sooner you start, the better!

Fit for Change

Where are you on the fitness continuum? You may already know that you need to cut back on calories, fat (especially saturated fat), cholesterol, or sodium. Or you may want to eat more complex carbohydrates, fiber, or certain vitamins and minerals. Or maybe overcoming a sedentary lifestyle is your challenge. No matter where you are now, you can benefit by charting your course toward achieving overall fitness.

Gradual changes for health are often easier and more effective in the long run than jumping in with leaps and bounds. So take it one month at a time—in fact, one *day* at a time.

Start by tracking your eating pattern and your physical activities over the next month. We've provided a month's worth of nutrition and activity record forms to chart your progress (see page 39). One month is long enough to see some results, but not too long to feel tedious. Use this day-by-day *Monthly Nutrition Companion* to help you...

➤ Become more aware of your personal eating and physical activity habits.

➤ Set short- and long-term fitness goals. And personalize a step-by-step action plan for healthful eating and physical activity.

➤ Monitor your weekly progress toward your goals and action plans for the month. Plus, spot your problem areas.

➤ Learn and acquire eating and physical activity habits that you can live with—for a lifetime of good health!

Keep in mind that change may require some "re-training." But, if you're motivated to live healthier, your investment of time and effort, as well as your personal motivation, will pay off!

Chapter Two

All About You

READY TO STEP TOWARD FITNESS? First, take a closer look at yourself—your current food decisions and your lifestyle.

Rate Your Plate

Think about your typical eating pattern and food decisions. Do you...

	Usually	Sometimes	Never
1. Consider nutrition when you make food choices?	❑	❑	❑
2. Try to eat regular meals (including breakfast), rather than skip or skimp on some?	❑	❑	❑
3. Choose nutritious snacks?	❑	❑	❑
4. Try to eat a variety of foods?	❑	❑	❑
5. Include new-to-you foods in meals and snacks?	❑	❑	❑
6. Try to balance your energy (calorie) intake with your physical activity?	❑	❑	❑

Now for the Details. Do You...

	Usually	Sometimes	Never
7. Eat at least 6 servings* of grain products daily?	❑	❑	❑
8. Eat at least 3 servings* of vegetables daily?	❑	❑	❑
9. Eat at least 2 servings* of fruits daily?	❑	❑	❑
10. Consume at least 2 servings* of milk, yogurt, or cheese daily?	❑	❑	❑

*Serving sizes vary depending on the food and food group. See pages 18 to 24 for specific examples.

11. Eat 2 servings* of meat, poultry, fish, beans, eggs, or nuts daily? ❏ ❏ ❏

12. Go easy on higher-fat foods? ❏ ❏ ❏

13. Go easy on sweets? ❏ ❏ ❏

14. Drink 8 or more cups of fluids daily? ❏ ❏ ❏

15. Limit alcoholic beverages (no more than 1 daily for a woman or 2 for a man)? ❏ ❏ ❏

Score yourself: 2 points for "usually," 1 point for "sometimes," and 0 points for "never." _____

If you scored:

24 to 30 points—Healthful eating seems to be your fitness habit already. Still, look for ways to stick to a healthful eating plan—and to make a "good thing" even better.

16 to 23 points—You're on track. A few easy changes could help you make your overall eating plan healthier.

9 to 15 points—Sometimes you eat smart—but not often enough to be your "fitness best." What might be your first steps to healthier eating?

0 to 8 points—For your good health, you're wise to rethink your overall eating style. Take it gradually—step by step!

Whatever your score, make moves for healthful eating. Gradually turn your "nevers" into "sometimes" and your "sometimes" into "usually."

Get in Touch

Consider: Why you eat what you do: when, where, and how? Do you...

(Check all that apply.)

1. Eat when you feel...?
   ❏ bored   ❏ stressed
   ❏ angry   ❏ lonely
   ❏ hungry   ❏ excited
   ❏ (other) _____

*Serving sizes vary depending on the food and food group. See pages 18 to 24 for specific examples.

Monthly Nutrition Companion

2. Eat when you are...?
- ❏ relaxing
- ❏ socializing with others
- ❏ (other) _____
- ❏ watching TV
- ❏ trying not to smoke

3. Eat meals and snacks in your...?
- ❏ kitchen
- ❏ family room
- ❏ deck/patio
- ❏ (other) _____
- ❏ dining room
- ❏ bedroom
- ❏ car

4. Typically eat...?
- ❏ breakfast
- ❏ dinner
- ❏ many mini meals
- ❏ lunch
- ❏ snack

5. Have an uncontrollable urge for some foods?
- ❏ yes
- ❏ no

If yes, jot down what typically triggers you to eat certain foods.

_____

_____

6. Let any obstacles get in the way of healthful eating?
- ❏ busy schedule
- ❏ habit
- ❏ cost
- ❏ conflicting or lack of or lack of information
- ❏ (other) _____
- ❏ not enough energy or motivation
- ❏ inconvenience
- ❏ don't want to give up taste
- ❏ no willpower

7. Buy meals away from home?
- ❏ yes
- ❏ no

If yes, how often in a typical week?_____ Where?
- ❏ quickservice (fast food) places
- ❏ buffets/all-you-can-eat restaurants
- ❏ table service restaurants
- ❏ delis/cafeterias
- ❏ sweet or dessert shops/coffee bars
- ❏ supermarket takeouts

For the previous questions, there are no right or wrong answers. Instead, they get you in touch with your eating style. And they help you set your action plans for healthful eating.

Check Your Weight

Weigh yourself: _____ pounds

Then find yourself on the chart below showing the healthy weight for adults of all ages. In each range, the higher weights usually apply to men and women with more muscle and a larger body frame.

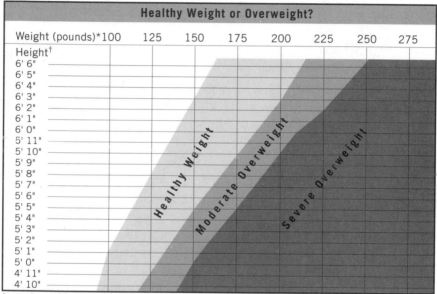

Source: *Report of the Dietary Guidelines Advisory Committee on the Dietary Guidelines for Americans, 1995.*
* without clothes
† without shoes

Where do you fit within the weight ranges?
- ☐ healthy weight
- ☐ overweight
- ☐ underweight

Figure Your Waist-to-Hip Ratio

Stand relaxed. Measure your waist at its smallest point. Don't tuck your stomach in..

Measure your hips at the largest part of your buttocks and hips.

Divide your waist measurement by hip measurement. For a healthy weight, most women should be below 0.80; for men, less than 0.95 is best.

Is your number nearly or more than 1.0? If so, your apple shape puts you at greater risk for some health problems, such as heart disease. If it's considerably less than 1.0, your pear shape makes extra weight less of an issue.

Rate Your "Gait"

Decide where your overall lifestyle and physical activity fit on this continuum. (Refer to page 15 for definitions of each level.)

1	2	3	4
Sedentary Activity	Light Activity	Moderate Activity	Very Active

If you're somewhere left of "moderate activity," even a small boost in your pace can offer added health benefits. Moderate physical activity offers many of the same benefits as more strenuous activity.

Now for the Details...

1. On average, how much time do you think you spend in physical activity:

   _____ minutes daily? _____ hours weekly?

2. What types of physical activities do you...

   enjoy? _____

   do often? _____

3. Do you include physical activities in your daily lifestyle, such as climbing stairs or housework?

   ❑ yes   ❑ no

   If yes, what? _____

   _____

4. What keeps you from getting enough physical activity? (Check any that apply.)

   ❑ busy schedule   ❑ cost
   ❑ lack of motivation   ❑ no energy
   ❑ inconvenience   ❑ (other)_____

   Whether it's active, everyday living or sports, health experts recommend at least 30 minutes of moderate physical activity on most, if not all, days of the week. If you come up short, you'll want to take steps toward a more active lifestyle. For more on what's considered moderate activity, refer to page 31.

Consider Change

Consider what you know about you—and what you know about fitness. Then check off the changes that you might make for a healthy life.

☐ Eat a greater variety of foods.

☐ Start the day with a nutritious meal.

☐ Consume more...*
  ☐ calcium   ☐ iron
  ☐ fiber   ☐ vitamin A
  ☐ vitamin C   ☐ other_____

☐ Consume less...*
  ☐ fat   ☐ saturated fat
  ☐ cholesterol   ☐ sodium
  ☐ other_____

☐ Eat more fruits and vegetables.

☐ Eat more breads and other grain products.

☐ Cut back on high-calorie, low-nutrient foods.

☐ Make nutritious snack choices.

☐ Lose _____ pounds.**

☐ Gain _____ pounds.**

☐ Get more physical activity.

☐ Other

_____

_____

* For foods that contain these nutrients and food substances, refer to pages 183 to 194.

** For guidance on setting a safe and effective action plan for weight management, refer to page 195.

How to Use Your *Monthly Nutrition Companion*

Using what you've learned about your food and activity habits, follow these easy steps to make your plan for smart eating and active living.

1. Start with a practical, sensible overview of healthful eating and physical activity. On pages 12 to 28 get to know the Food Guide Pyramid and physical activity guidelines and how they apply to your life. When you need to know more, refer to pages 181 to 199.

2. Set personal goals. Then make a step-by-step action plan. Pages 29 to 34 are your personal planning guide. Set realistic goals and make changes gradually. Small changes add up over time.

3. Track your progress. Use the day-by-day eating and physical activity record, starting on page 39. If you get off track, pick up where you left off, and start again.

4. Reward your successes along the way. As you complete "Your Weekly Check-Up," pat yourself on the back. Change deserves recognition!

5. At the end of the month, evaluate your progress, and reevaluate your plan on page 178. Revisit this questionnaire, too. See how you've moved toward fitness—and decide your next steps.

Here's to your health!

Chapter Three

Eating for Fitness!

HEALTHY EATING is all about what's right for you. And it's about making healthful choices that fit your lifestyle—so that you can do things that matter to you.

What are the basics of healthful eating? Dietary Guidelines for Americans offer bottom-line advice. Whatever your age, gender, or lifestyle, these seven guidelines represent the most current thinking of today's health professionals. And they're based on sound science.

The Dietary Guidelines are meant to help all healthy people, ages two and over, make food choices that help maintain, and perhaps improve, health.

Nutrition and Your Health:
Dietary Guidelines for Americans

- ➤ Eat a variety of foods.
- ➤ Balance the food you eat with physical activity—maintain or improve your weight.
- ➤ Choose a diet with plenty of grain products, vegetables, and fruits.
- ➤ Choose a diet low in fat, saturated fat, and cholesterol.
- ➤ Choose a diet moderate in sugars.
- ➤ Choose a diet moderate in salt and sodium.
- ➤ If you drink alcoholic beverages, do so in moderation.

Source: U.S. Department of Agriculture/ U.S. Department of Health and Human Services, 1995.

While these guidelines may sound a bit daunting, they can be easy to put into action. Healthful eating, as part of a healthy lifestyle, takes your personal commitment. In fact, "It's All About You" and what you want out of life.

Make healthful choices that fit your lifestyle so that you can do the things you want to do.

Be realistic. Make small changes over time in what you eat and the level of activity you do. After all, small steps work better than giant leaps.

Be adventurous. Expand your tastes to enjoy a variety of foods.

Be flexible. Go ahead and balance what you eat and the physical activity you do over several days. There's no need to worry about just one meal or one day.

Be sensible. Enjoy all foods, just don't overdo it.

Be active. Remember, walk the dog, don't just watch the dog walk!

Source: Dietary Guidelines Alliance, 1996.

Pyramid Your Way to Healthful Eating

Planning for healthful eating is like building a pyramid—with five nutrient-filled building blocks as the base, and a small pyramid tip with fats, oils, and sweets. No matter what your lifestyle, the Food Guide Pyramid is your personal eating guide. It's an action plan that turns the Dietary Guidelines into a strategy for healthful eating.

The Food Guide Pyramid is designed for all healthy people—male or female, young or old—ages two and above. Because it's so flexible, use it to choose foods that match your lifestyle and your food preferences. Good news: all foods fit into a healthful eating plan!

Food Guide Pyramid

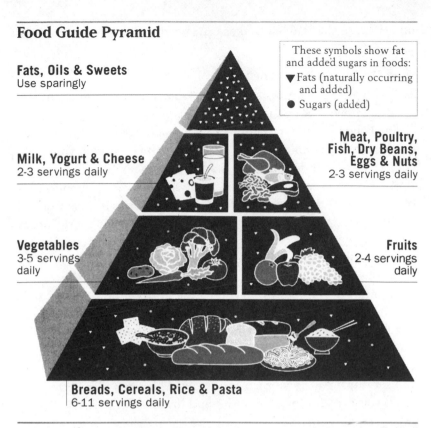

Fats, Oils & Sweets
Use sparingly

These symbols show fat and added sugars in foods:
▼ Fats (naturally occurring and added)
● Sugars (added)

Milk, Yogurt & Cheese
2-3 servings daily

Meat, Poultry, Fish, Dry Beans, Eggs & Nuts
2-3 servings daily

Vegetables
3-5 servings daily

Fruits
2-4 servings daily

Breads, Cereals, Rice & Pasta
6-11 servings daily

Variety, balance, and moderation: that's how the Pyramid defines healthful eating.

Variety means...eating different foods—both within the five food groups and among them. After all, no one food or food group supplies all the nutrients your body needs. Variety makes eating more fun, too!

Balance means...eating enough, but not too much, from each food group daily. The range of servings suggests how much.

Moderation means...controlling the calories and the total amount of fat, saturated fat, cholesterol, sodium, sugars, and, if consumed, alcoholic beverages. For example, opt mostly for low-fat and lean choices within each food group. And go easy on foods (from the Pyramid tip) that supply energy, or calories, but few nutrients.

Whatever your typical daily eating pattern—three meals, perhaps with snacks, or several mini-meals—Pyramid guidelines apply. Read

Eating for Fitness!

on for more about what makes up a serving size from each Pyramid group.

How Much Is Enough—For You?

To follow the Pyramid's advice for balance and moderation, you need to know about servings: how many and what size.

The Food Guide Pyramid recommends a range of servings, not a single amount, from each food group to help you match your food choices to your individual needs and preferences.

For enough nutrients, Pyramid guidelines advise everyone—ages two and over—to consume at least the minimum servings from all five food groups on most days. Beyond that, different energy needs dictate how many servings are best. Energy needs depend on age, gender, health, and level of physical activity.

Do the serving ranges seem like a lot of food? Actually, eating the minimum number of servings from all five food groups adds up to only about 1,600 calories—if the choices are mostly lean and low-fat foods. That's about right for many inactive women and older adults. Others may need more.

Here's how three energy, or calorie, targets can be met with Pyramid servings. Your own plan for Pyramid servings may differ, but you'll want to aim for at least the "minimums."

	Less Active Women,* Older Adults	Children,** Teen Girls, Active Women,* Less Active Men	Teen Boys, Active Men
Calories	about 1,600	about 2,200	about 2,800
Bread Group	6	9	11
Vegetable Group	3	4	5
Fruit Group	2	3	4
Milk Group***	2-3	2-3	2-3
Meat Group	2 (5 oz. total)	2 (6 oz. total)	3 (7 oz. total)

*Pregnancy and breast-feeding may require more calories.

**Preschool children may need less than 1,600 calories daily. Except for milk, smaller servings are appropriate to meet their energy needs.

***Women who are pregnant or breast-feeding, teenagers, and young adults to age 24 need at least three servings.

How Many Servings per Day?

Follow the Pyramid guidelines for the number of servings you should aim for on most days of the week. It's OK if you eat more or less on some days—your food choices over time are what counts. Keep in mind that the serving amounts suggested on the previous page are based on mostly low-fat and lean food choices with moderate amounts of fats, oils, and sweets.

Just for You

Servings: Enough, Not Too Much. How much energy your body uses will determine how many food group servings you need. Use the following five steps to make a quick guess-timate of your daily energy needs. Determine:

1. Your basic energy needs: energy to keep your body processes going—for example, your heartbeat, breathing, regulating body temperature, and sending messages to your brain.

_____ pounds (your healthy weight) x _____*

= _____ your calories for basic needs

*Multiply by 10 for women and by 11 for men.

Example: 135 pounds x 10 (for woman) =
1,350 calories for basic energy needs

2. Your energy needs for physical activity: Check the activity that matches your typical lifestyle:

❏ **Sedentary activity:** mainly sitting, standing, reading, typing, or other low-intensity activities

❏ **Light activity:** such as walking, for no more than 2 hours daily

❏ **Moderate activity:** such as heavy housework, gardening, dancing, brisk walking, and very little sitting

❏ **Very active:** labor-intensive job, such as construction work or ditch digging, or active physical sports, such as running or basketball

Multiply your basic energy needs by the percent that matches your activity level: sedentary—20%, light—30%, moderate—40%, or very active—50%.

_____ calories for basic needs

x _____ % for activity level

= _____ your calories for physical activity

Example: 1,350 calories for basic needs

x 0.30 for light activity

= 405 calories for physical activity

3. Your energy needs for digestion and absorbing nutrients:

0.10 x (_____ calories for basic needs

+ _____ calories for physical activity)

= _____ your calories for digestion
and absorbing nutrients

Example: 0.10 x (1,350 calories for basic needs

+ 405 calories for physical activity)

= 175.5 calories

4. Your overall energy needs:

_____ calories for basic needs

+ _____ calories for physical activity

+ _____ calories for digestion and absorbing
nutrients

= _____ your overall energy, or calorie, needs

Example:

1,350 calories for basic needs

+ 405 calories for activity

+ 176 calories for digestion and
absorbing nutrients (rounded)

= 1,931 overall calories (approximate)

5. Your personal Pyramid: Compare your overall energy needs to the calorie levels in chart on page 14. If your needs fall between calorie levels, approximate the number of servings based on the calorie level closest to your needs. Write how many food group servings you might consume daily to meet your needs.

Bread Group   _____ servings

Vegetable Group   _____ servings

Fruit Group   _____ servings

Milk Group   _____ servings

Meat Group   _____ servings

What counts as a serving? The amount depends on the food and the food group. Look for examples on pages 18 to 24. "Sizing It All Up" on page 26 shows how to estimate serving sizes.

Your Foods—Where Do They Fit?

Think of any food or beverage you've ever had, including your favorites. Whatever the food, it fits somewhere in the Food Guide Pyramid—either in one food group, or in several food groups if it's a mixed or combo food, or in the Pyramid tip. In fact, all foods can fit!

Why are foods grouped together—and what do foods in each food group have in common? Their nutrient content is similar, therefore they promote your health in comparable ways. Each food group supplies some, but not all, nutrients you need for health. That's why choosing a variety of foods, both within and among the food groups, is so important.

Just for You

Something old, something new. Jot down five of your favorite foods, plus two or three foods you'd like to try. Where do they fit on the Food Guide Pyramid?

Your Food Favorites   **Food Group(s)**

_____   _____

_____   _____

_____   _____

_____   _____

New-to-You Foods   **Food Group(s)**

_____   _____

_____   _____

_____   _____

Not sure where these foods fit inside the Pyramid, or how they promote your good health? Read on for guidance.

Bread, Cereal, Rice, and Pasta Group

Inside the Pyramid... Bread Group foods are made from grains: barley, buckwheat, bulgur, corn, oats, quinoa, rice, rye, wheat, among others. These grains may be ground into flour for breads, other baked goods, dumplings, pasta, pancakes, tortillas, wonton wrappers, pretzels, and other foods. Some are eaten as cooked cereals—for example, rice and grits—and as ready-to-eat breakfast cereals.

Their nutrient contribution... Foods made from grains supply complex carbohydrates—your main energy source—and B vitamins. Among other functions, B vitamins help your body use energy. Whole-grain and enriched grain products supply iron; among its roles, iron helps your blood carry oxygen to body cells for energy production. Whole-grain foods are good sources of fiber, which aids digestion and may help protect you from heart disease and some cancers. Most Bread Group foods are low in fat.

For more on the fat and fiber content of certain Bread Group foods, refer to pages 184 and 192 to 193.

Your Bread Group servings... 6 to 11 servings daily.

A serving is...
- ➤ 1 slice (1 oz.) enriched or whole-grain bread
- ➤ 1/2 hamburger roll, bagel, English muffin, or pita
- ➤ 1 (6-inch) tortilla
- ➤ 1/2 cup cooked rice or pasta
- ➤ 1/2 cup cooked oatmeal, grits, barley, or cream of wheat cereal
- ➤ 1/2 cup quinoa, bulgur, millet, or other whole grain
- ➤ 1 ounce (1 cup) ready-to-eat cereal
- ➤ 3 to 4 small crackers
- ➤ 1 (4-inch) diameter pancake or waffle
- ➤ 3 tablespoons wheat germ
- ➤ 2 medium cookies

Pyramid pointers...
- ➤ Boost "carbs" by putting pasta, rice, or other grain foods center stage at your meal or snack.
- ➤ To "fiber up," eat at least three whole-grain foods a day.
- ➤ Opt for breads made with less fat and sugars, such as

bagels, bread sticks, pita bread, and English muffins. Go easy on those with more fat or sugars, such as croissants, doughnuts, and sweet rolls.

➤ Try Bread Group foods that may be new to you: perhaps amaranth, couscous, quinoa, or millet. Or try a different grain-based dish: risotto, polenta, or tabouli.

Vegetable Group

Inside the Pyramid... From A to Z—arugula to zucchini—there's a wide array of foods in the Vegetable Group. Legumes have a split personality; they fit in both the Vegetable Group and the Meat Group, but can't count as servings toward both.

Their nutrient contribution... Nutritionally speaking, vegetables vary; that's why choosing a variety makes health-sense.

Deep yellow and dark green leafy vegetables, such as carrots, sweet potatoes, kale, spinach, and broccoli, are good sources of beta carotene, which forms vitamin A. Among its other jobs, vitamin A helps keep your eyes and skin healthy. Antioxidant properties of beta carotene may offer protection from some ongoing diseases.

Other vegetables, such as brussels sprouts, bell peppers, cabbages, and tomatoes, are good sources of vitamin C. Vitamin C has many functions, including helping your body use iron from plant sources of food and resist infection. Vitamin C also acts as an antioxidant perhaps offering protection from some ongoing health problems.

Vegetables supply other essential vitamins, including folic acid. Folic acid, especially important for women who are pregnant or planning to get pregnant, helps reduce the risk of birth defects.

While most vegetables have few calories and little fat, many are good sources of complex carbohydrates, your body's main energy source. And many are good fiber sources.

For more on the vitamin A, vitamin C, and fiber content of certain Vegetable Group foods, refer to pages 187 to 189 and 192.

Your Vegetable Group servings... 3 to 5 servings daily.

A serving is...
➤ 1/2 cup chopped raw, nonleafy vegetables
➤ 1 cup leafy raw vegetables (lettuce, spinach, watercress, cabbage)

- ➤ 1/2 cup cooked vegetables
- ➤ 1/2 cup cooked legumes
- ➤ 1 small baked potato (3 ounces)
- ➤ 3/4 cup vegetable juice

Pyramid pointers...

- ➤ Eat many different types of vegetables because they have varying amounts and types of nutrients.
- ➤ Try to eat dark green leafy and deep yellow vegetables (red, orange, and yellow) every day: for example, collard greens, spinach, red bell pepper, tomato, and sweet potatoes. They supply carotenoids, such as beta carotene, which form vitamin A in your body.
- ➤ For more fiber, keep edible peels on vegetables such as potatoes, cucumber, and summer squash.
- ➤ Broaden your personal vegetable menu beyond favorite standbys. Perhaps try brussels sprouts, chard, kale, parsnips, beets, bok choy, okra, and various squashes.
- ➤ Enjoy the vegetables you've always eaten—just eat more of them.

Fruit Group

Inside the Pyramid... All kinds of fruits can fill your "fruit bowl." Fruit juices as well as dried fruits, such as dried apricots, dates, and raisins, fit in the Fruit Group, too.

Their nutrient contribution... Like vegetables, fruits supply varying amounts of vitamins A and C, as well as other nutrients. Citrus fruits (orange, grapefruit, tangerine), melons, and berries are excellent sources of vitamin C. And many deep yellow fruits, such as apricots, cantaloupe, mangoes, and peaches, are good vitamin A sources.

Fruits supply simple carbohydrates, or sugars, which provide energy. Like many vegetables, some provide folate, as well as fiber (especially with the edible peels on). And many provide potassium, which helps regulate body fluids and maintain your blood pressure.

For more on the vitamin A, vitamin C, and fiber content of certain Fruit Group foods, refer to pages 187 to 189 and 192.

Your Fruit Group servings... 2 to 4 servings daily.

A serving is...
- ➤ 1 medium fruit (apple, orange, banana, peach)
- ➤ 1/2 grapefruit, mango, or papaya
- ➤ 3/4 cup fruit juice
- ➤ 1/2 cup berries or cut-up fruit
- ➤ 1/2 cup canned, frozen, or cooked fruit
- ➤ 1/4 cup dried fruit

Pyramid pointers...
- ➤ Every day, try to include a vitamin-C rich fruit or fruit juice among your food choices: perhaps citrus fruit, berries, or melon. Breakfast is a great opportunity!
- ➤ Drink fruit juice as a snack beverage.
- ➤ Keep dried fruits—raisins, prunes, dried apricots, dried apple slices, dried cranberries—handy for healthful nibbling and pack-and-go meals and snacks.
- ➤ Go beyond the basics with less common fruits, such as figs, kiwifruit, lychee, mango, papaya, or prickly pear.
- ➤ To sweeten your palate, eat fruit for dessert!

Milk, Yogurt, and Cheese Group

Inside the Pyramid... Foods from the Milk Group include milk itself (whole, 2%, low-fat, and fat-free) as well as foods made from milk: yogurt, hard cheese, ricotta and cottage cheese, frozen yogurt, ice cream, milk shake, and pudding. Although calcium-fortified soy milk isn't made from milk, it belongs here, too.

Their nutrient contribution... Milk Group foods supply many nutrients, especially protein, calcium, and riboflavin. Among other jobs, calcium helps bones grow and stay strong and healthy. And protein, a part of every body cell, is needed to build and maintain healthy body tissue.

The fat content varies within the Milk Group; fat-free, low-fat (1%), and reduced-fat (2%) milk products have less fat than whole-milk products. Cheese may be full-fat, reduced-fat, or fat-free.

For more on the fat and calcium in certain Milk Group foods, refer to pages 185 and 189 to 190.

Your Milk Group servings... 2 to 3 servings daily.

A serving is...

➤ 1 cup milk, buttermilk, or yogurt
➤ 1/2 cup evaporated milk
➤ 1/3 cup dry milk
➤ 1 1/2 ounces natural cheese (cheddar, mozzarella, Swiss, Monterey Jack)
➤ 1/2 cup ricotta cheese
➤ 2 ounces process cheese (American)

Count as 1/2 serving:

➤ 1/2 cup frozen yogurt
➤ 1 cup cottage cheese

Count as 1/3 serving:

➤ 1/2 cup ice cream

Pyramid pointers...

➤ Start your day with dairy: perhaps yogurt, a yogurt-fruit smoothie, or milk on cereal.
➤ Look for easy add-ons: shredded cheese on soups or salads, yogurt dips with veggies, milk in coffee or tea, or cheese on sandwiches.
➤ Make calcium-rich dairy foods your snacktime choices: perhaps cheese cubes, yogurt, milk, frozen yogurt, or pudding.
➤ Order a carton of milk to go with your deli or quickservice meals.

Meat, Poultry, Fish, Beans, Eggs, and Nuts Group

Inside the Pyramid... Foods in this group are a mixed bag, some from animal sources, others from plant sources. The common denominator is that they're all good protein sources. All kinds of meat (beef, pork, lamb, game meat), poultry, fish, and eggs belong in the Meat Group. So do legumes (beans, peas, and lentils), nuts, and seeds. Foods made from legumes fit here, too: for example, tofu, refried beans, and peanut butter.

Their nutrient contribution... Meat Group foods are high in protein, as well as iron, zinc, and some B vitamins. Iron helps carry oxygen to cells, where it's used to produce energy. Among other roles, zinc helps build and repair body cells and tissues. Legumes also contain both complex carbohydrates and fiber.

Unless they're prepared with fat, lower-fat choices from the Meat Group include lean meat, poultry without skin, seafood, and beans. Nuts and seeds have more fat.

For more on the fat, iron, and fiber in certain Meat Group foods, refer to pages 185 to 186, 190 to 191, and 191 to 193.

Your Meat Group servings... 2 to 3 servings (5 to 7 ounces total) daily.

A serving is...
- 2 to 3 ounces cooked lean meat, poultry, or fish; or sliced lean deli meat; or canned tuna or salmon

Count as 1 ounce meat:
- 1/2 cup cooked legumes
- 1 egg
- 1/4 cup egg substitute
- 2 tablespoons peanut butter
- 1/3 cup nuts
- 4 ounces tofu

Count as 2 ounces meat:
- 1/2 cup tuna or ground beef
- 1 small chicken leg or thigh
- 2 slices sandwich-size meat

Count as 3 ounces meat:
- 1 medium pork chop
- 1/4 pound hamburger patty (raw weight)
- 1/2 chicken breast
- 1 unbreaded 3-ounce fish filet

Pyramid pointers...
- Consider the size of your Meat Group portions. Five to seven ounces a day provides enough protein for most people.
- Choose egg-based dishes occasionally. To avoid too much cholesterol, consume no more than four egg yolks per week, including yolks in prepared foods.

Eating for Fitness!

- Feature legumes in meals: perhaps in tacos or burritos, salads, soups, stews, pasta sauces, stir-fries, or as potato toppers. Beans, peas, and lentils are low in fat and packed with protein, complex carbohydrate, and fiber!
- Try to eat seafood several times a week. It has less total fat and saturated fat than meat or poultry, and contains omega-three fatty acids, which may help protect you from heart disease.
- Use tofu, tempeh, and textured soy protein—all made from soybeans—in stir-fries, casseroles, soups, and other dishes.

Fats, Oils, and Sweets

Inside the Pyramid tip... Foods with high proportions of naturally occurring or added fats or with added sugars fit mostly within the Pyramid tip: salad dressings, oils, cream, butter, margarine, cream cheese, gravy, sugars, soft drinks, jams and jellies, sherbet, and gelatin desserts.

Their nutrient contribution... These foods or food ingredients contribute fat or sugars. So they supply mostly calories, but few, if any, other nutrients. For more on the fat content of foods, refer to page 184 to 187.

Just a bit from the Pyramid tip... There are no recommended serving sizes or ranges for these foods. Just eat them sparingly. In small amounts, they add flavor and pleasure to your meals and snacks.

Pyramid pointers...

- Go easy on spreads, salad dressings, toppings, gravies, and sauces that add fat or sugars to foods.
- Enjoy soft drinks and candies in moderation.
- Go easy on cream cheese, sour cream, and margarine—or try low-fat varieties. Cream cheese and sour cream are also sold in fat-free versions.

What a Great Combo!

A slice of bread or a piece of fruit is easy to classify into a food group. But where do lasagna, pizza, quiche, or a chef's salad fit?

It's easy to decide if you start with the main ingredients. Combination foods, which are made with several ingredients, may offer full or partial servings from several food groups. You need to "take apart" the dish to decide just how many. As an example, see how two chicken fajitas are classified.

Two Chicken Fajitas

Ingredient	Amount	Food Group	Servings
Chicken	2 oz.	Meat	2/3 to 1
Salsa	4 Tbsp.	Vegetable	1/2
Bell pepper and onions	1/2 c.	Vegetable	1
Cheese shreds	3 Tbsp.	Milk	1/2
Sour cream	2 tsp.	Fats, Oils, Sweets	NA*
Soft tortilla	2 (6-inch)	Bread	2

* NA = not applicable. There are no recommended servings from the Pyramid tip; just eat them sparingly.

· ·

Just for You

Take It Apart. Now, what combo food do you enjoy eating? Just for practice, decide where it fits within the Pyramid and then determine how many servings a typical portion gives you. Use serving information on pages 18 to 24 to help you.

Your combo food _____

Ingredient	Amount	Food Group Serving

· ·

Sizing It All Up

To use the Pyramid, with its five food groups, as your planning guide, you need to know what counts as one serving. A slightly bigger portion may count as more than one serving; a smaller portion, as just a partial serving.

From food group to food group, and from food to food, you likely noticed that serving sizes differ a bit. Pages 18 to 24 give examples of serving sizes within each of the five food groups.

Judging your own servings may take practice. How much, for example, is a 3-ounce serving of meat or 1 1/2 ounces of cheese? Use these visual comparisons to make quick guess-timates of your serving sizes:

This serving...	Is about the size of...
3 ounces of meat, poultry, or fish	deck of playing cards
1 ounce of meat, poultry, or fish	matchbox
1 cup fruit, yogurt	baseball
1/2 cup pasta, rice, fruit, or vegetables	1/2 baseball or tennis ball
1 medium potato	computer mouse
1 medium orange, peach, or apple	tennis ball
1 average bagel	hockey puck
1 cup chopped fresh leafy greens	4 lettuce leaves
2 Tbsp. peanut butter	Ping-Pong ball
1 ounce cheese*	four dice

* 1 ounce of brick or sliced cheese makes 1/4 cup shredded cheese.

Tip: Even low-calorie, low-fat, and fat-free foods can add up to a hefty calorie count when portions get large.

Just for You

It's Your Serve! Do your portions count as one Pyramid serving, or a little more or less? Next time you pour a bowl of cereal or serve a portion of rice or pasta, measure it. Or weigh your burger patty on a kitchen scale. You may be surprised. Your portions may be bigger, or smaller, than you think!

Good news: Once you have a feel for portion sizes, you don't need to weigh or measure your food choices. Serving sizes are just general guides. Try to come close to the recommended totals, on average, over several days.

Fluid Assets

Do you "thirst for success"? Then drink enough fluids. For good health, you need at least 8 cups of water daily—from drinking water, other beverages, and water in solid foods. That's to replace what your body loses daily as you perspire, eliminate body wastes, and breathe. With strenuous activity and hot, humid weather, you may need more.

Water is, after all, an essential nutrient required for many body functions. It makes up 55 to 75 percent of your weight. Without enough, you may get dehydrated. Fluid loss can lead to weakness, breathing problems, higher temperature and pulse rates, heat exhaustion, and even heatstroke.

Hint: Caffeinated drinks and alcoholic beverages may not provide as much fluid replacement benefit as you might think. They have a diuretic effect, increasing fluid loss through urination. Get most of your fluids from beverages without caffeine or alcohol.

On their own, alcoholic beverages offer little nutritionally—except for calories. And in excess, their alcohol can pose health and accident risks. A moderate amount—no more than 1 drink (12 ounces beer, or 5 ounces wine, or 1 1/2 ounces liquor) a day for women, and 2 for men—is OK for most healthy people.

Drops of Wisdom...

➤ For great fluid sources, drink fruit and vegetable juices, milk, buttermilk, soup—or just plain water!

➤ "Water down" meals and snacks with water, milk, or juice. Or try yogurt-juice drinks.

➤ Walking by a water fountain? Take a drink.

➤ Sip as you work? Keep a cup of water on your desk. Or reach for boxed or canned juice.

➤ Before, during, and after physical activity—drink plenty of fluids.

➤ Refresh yourself with sparkling water or juice as your party drink of choice.

Just for You

Enough Fluids? On weekends or days when you're home, try this. In the morning, fill a jug with 8 cups of water. Put it in the fridge. Then use it as drinking water or for making juice, lemonade, soup, tea, or coffee. When the water is gone, you've likely met your fluid goal for the day.

Chapter Four

Making Your
Best Moves

WHETHER YOU'RE INVOLVED IN SPORTS, or simply live an active lifestyle, physical activity is your right move for fitness. Physical activity and healthful eating go hand in hand with good health.

Get Moving: For Health-Smart Reasons!

No time or opportunity? Think again. You can't afford to neglect regular physical activity. Consider the health dividends of regular, moderate physical activity!

Leaner, trimmer body... easier to lose weight and keep it off.

Less risk for health problems... including heart disease, diabetes, high blood pressure, high blood cholesterol levels, osteoporosis, and some cancers.

Stronger bones, less risk of fractures... if weight-bearing exercise (walking, running, weight-lifting, others) is part of your routine.

Stronger muscles... for sports and everyday activities such as moving, carrying, and lifting things. As you build more muscle, the rate your body uses energy goes up, too. That's a benefit for weight management.

Healthier heart... to pump blood and nutrients more easily through your 60,000 miles of blood vessels.

More endurance... during physical activity and for increased stamina overall. That may boost your productivity!

Injury protection... allowing you to move away from pending danger faster...or more easily catch yourself if you slip or trip.

Better coordination and flexibility... allowing you to move with greater ease and range of motion.

Feel younger longer... by slowing some signs of aging.

Stress relief, better sleep... allowing your body to relax and release emotional tension, and helping you sleep better.

Better mental outlook... which may boost your feeling of well-being and give you an energizing attitude!

Bonus reason: why not? A physically active lifestyle can be fun!

How to Get Moving

Variety, balance, and moderation are guidelines for physical activity—as they are for healthful eating. For your good health:

Enjoy a **variety** of activities to exercise different parts of your body—including your heart! They might be everyday tasks such as gardening or your favorite sport.

Balance your physical activities to get different benefits, for example:
> bone strength (walking, strength training, and other weight-bearing activities)
> flexibility (stretching and bending activities)
> muscle strength (weight training, tennis, calisthenics)
> cardiovascular endurance (brisk walking, square dancing, lap swimming, jumping rope, other aerobic activities)

Stay fit with physical activity that's right for you, without overdoing. Try to fit **moderate** activity into your daily routine. That means 30 minutes or more a day, on most, if not all, days of the week. More rigorous, sustained activities offer extra benefits for cardiovascular, or heart, health.

What is a moderate level of physical activity? It's the amount that uses up about 150 calories a day, or about 1,000 calories a week. Meet this goal with one longer activity, or mix and match several shorter activities over the course of one day.

Each of the everyday tasks or sports on the next page could add up to a moderate level of activity for a day.

What is Moderate Activity?

	Minutes	less vigorous, more time
Washing and waxing a car	45-60	
Washing windows or floors	45-60	
Playing volleyball	45	
Playing touch football	30-45	
Gardening	30-45	
Wheeling self in wheelchair	30-40	
Walking 1 3/4 miles (20-minute mile)	35	
Basketball (shooting baskets)	30	
Bicycling 5 miles	30	
Dancing fast (social)	30	
Pushing a stroller 1 1/2 miles	30	
Raking leaves	30	
Walking 2 miles (15-minute mile)	30	
Water aerobics	30	
Swimming laps	20	
Wheelchair basketball	20	
Basketball (playing a game)	15-20	
Bicycling 4 miles	15	
Jumping rope	15	
Running 1 1/2 miles (10-minute mile)	15	
Shoveling snow	15	more vigorous, less time
Stairwalking	15	

Source: *Report of the Surgeon General*, U.S. Department of Health and Human Services, Centers for Disease Control and Prevention, The President's Council on Physical Fitness and Sports, 1996.

• •

Just for You

Your Best Moves. Write five ways—everyday tasks or sports—you might include moderate physical activity in your daily routine. These may be activities you already do, or they may be new to you.

What activities?   **How long?**

1. _____

2. _____

3. _____

4. _____

5. _____

• •

Making Your Best Moves

Chapter Five
Charting
Your Course

SET YOURSELF UP FOR SUCCESS. For healthful eating and an active
lifestyle, these strategies can help you get fit for a longer, healthier life.

Build Your Pyramid for Fitness
**Take stock of your everyday food choices—foods you eat at home and
away.** Identify your strong and weak points: what you eat, when,
where, with whom, and why. Refer to "All About You" on page 3.
By starting a food record on page 46, you'll learn even more!

Modify your food choices step by step. Be realistic. Rather than over-
haul your whole way of eating at one time, start small: perhaps one
more vegetable at dinner, less salad dressing, a switch to whole-grain
bread, a fruit snack, or a better breakfast. As you achieve small goals,
make more changes. Look for the healthy eating tips on each food
record page for small steps you might take.

Follow Pyramid advice. Choose from all five food groups daily, with
plenty of grain products, vegetables, fruits, as well as calcium-rich
dairy foods and protein-rich meat and meat alternates.

Make moderation your goal. You can eat what you like—no need to
give up your food favorites. Just choose nutrient-filled, high-fiber,
low-fat foods more often than their less healthful counterparts.

Choose variety within and among the food groups for their different
nutritional benefits and for the pleasure that variety adds to meals
and snacks.

Practice the fine art of balance, enough from each food group, but not too much.

Give snacks status on your personal Pyramid. Choose mostly those that contribute food-group servings!

"Rate your plate" by looking at the big picture; what you eat for several days, not one meal or one day.

Match food choices to your lifestyle. Avoid overdoing or underdoing on calories. Choose enough food-group servings to achieve and maintain your healthy weight.

Ask an expert. If you need guidance on healthful eating before you start—or as you go along—contact a registered dietitian or other qualified nutrition expert. See page 199.

Get Smart, Get Set, Get Moving!

Start with a physical exam, especially if you're over age 40, overweight, or have a heart, circulation, joint, or bone problem.

Assess your current level of physical activity—what you do, when, and how much. Refer back to your responses in "All About You" on page 3. Then keep the physical activity record, along with your food record, to see how active you really are.

Find a variety of activities you enjoy; not necessarily elaborate or expensive ones, just ones you'll stick with. And choose those that give you different benefits.

Start slowly. Take it one step at a time. For overall fitness, you need a total of 30 minutes or more of moderate activity most, if not all, days of the week. Smaller increments are OK: perhaps 15 minutes of lunch-hour walking plus 15 minutes of playing Frisbee with the kids later.

Build up to longer, more intense activity over a month or two—or even more—as you're ready. That builds cardiovascular fitness. Over time, you might add new or different activities to your repertoire.

Warm up and cool down—to prevent injury and improve performance with activities for building endurance and strength.

Make time! Adjust your schedule so that physical activity becomes a habit and part of your daily routine.

Choose activities that fit your day—with what you can and will do! Consider convenience so that your activity plan is easy for you to keep up.

Need motivation? Get fit with a friend! Or join a group, perhaps for tennis or line dancing, that meets regularly. As activity becomes routine, motivation comes from within—that's your true mark of success!

See how far you've come. Rather than think about sore muscles, focus on how good you feel: more energetic, less stressed, better mood, even better sleep.

Stepping to Fitness:
Your Personal Goals and Action Plans

Consider what you've learned about yourself from the questionnaire on page 3 and the "Just for You" sections. Now set your own goals and action plans, step-by-step, for healthful eating, physical activity, and lifelong health!

Your day's goals for Pyramid servings (Refer to pages 15 to 17.)

	Servings
Bread Group	_____
Vegetable Group	_____
Fruit Group	_____
Milk Group	_____
Meat Group	_____

For healthful eating...

Your Personal Goals	Your Reasons	Your Action Plans
For example:		
Eat more calcium-rich foods.	For healthy bones	Order milk with fast food meals. Pack yogurt in my lunch.
My cholesterol level is 235 mg/dL; my goal, 190 mg/dL.	For heart health	Make cereal and low-fat milk my typical breakfast; opt for eggs and bacon only occasionally.

For physical activity…

Your Personal Goals	Your Reasons	Your Action Plans
For example:		
Make weight-bearing exercise part of my daily routine.	For healthy bones	Walk during lunch break. Use the steps at work.
Lower my cholesterol level to 190 mg/dL.	For heart health	Ride my stationary bike. Start with 10 min. daily.

For both healthful eating and physical activity, circle the goals and action plans from the preceding pages that you'll start the first week. Remember, small steps work better than giant leaps!

Write down some rewards for making these changes...

For example:

Buy walking shoes for my walking routine

_____

_____

_____

_____

_____

_____

_____

_____

_____

_____

_____

_____

_____

_____

_____

_____

_____

_____

Sign On!

Now, make these goals and action plans your personal contract for fitness.

_____   _____
(Your signature)   (Date)

Chapter Six

Your Day-by-Day Companion

TRACKING YOUR FOOD and physical activity pattern can help you be more successful in your step-by-step approach to healthful living. This record book is flexible to match your needs. Keep eating and activity records for 4 weeks (28 days), starting on any day you choose. Or keep track for an entire month. (Day 1 starts on page 46.)

How do you keep the records? First keep this *Monthly Nutrition Companion* with you—wherever you go. Record your day's food and beverage choices (and the circumstances) and your physical activities right away. Then you won't need to recall your day later on.

Then, after each week, use your Weekly Check-Up to see how healthful eating and physical activity are becoming part of your daily routine, to spot your problem areas, and to set small goals and action plans for next week. For each week's successes, give yourself a non-food reward!

At the end of the month, use your Monthly Check-Up to see where you stand after the month—and to plan your next steps toward fitness!

Keeping a Daily Food Record

Start with the date. Then record everything you eat and drink from the time you wake up to the time you go to sleep.

Time. Record the time for meals, snacks, even beverage breaks.

Place. Write in the place you eat—perhaps the kitchen, in front of the TV, in the car, or at your desk.

Food and Beverage. Write down everything you eat and drink. Be specific about the kinds and amounts of food, including milk in your coffee and margarine on your toast, and about how food was prepared.

Amount. Estimate your portion sizes. Use the serving size guide on page 26 to help judge serving sizes.

Food Group/Servings. Decide what food group your food and drinks belong in, and how many food-group servings they contribute. Remember, some foods may be combo foods; refer to page 24 to help you fit them within the food groups.

Social Situation. Record who you were with and what were you doing. Social situations can influence food choices.

Hunger Level. Rate your hunger level each time you eat: "very hungry" = 3, "somewhat hungry" = 2, "not hungry" = 1.

Comments. Jot down how you feel (frustrated, bored, happy), your thoughts (lonely to eat alone, nice to eat with friends), or concerns (stressed at work).

For an example, see pages 42 and 43.

Checking Your Daily Pyramid

At the end of each day, give yourself a Pyramid check-up. Inside each of the five food groups on the empty Pyramid, record the total number of servings that you consumed for the day. Then answer the quick questions that follow. For an example, see page 44.

Keeping a Physical Activity Record

Day by day, track the ways you fit physical activity into your daily schedule.

Time of Day. Record the time of day.

Type of Physical Activity. That includes those physical activities of moderate to very active intensity: everyday activities (walking the dog, heavy gardening, or playing actively with your kids) or any physical activities (biking, jogging, or tennis). Refer to page 31 and the tips throughout the record for more examples of everyday physical activities.

Intensity. Rate your activity: "very active" = 4 and "moderately active" = 3.

Time Spent. Record the duration of your activity. Don't count light or sedentary activities, which are rated as 2 or 1, respectively. Then add up your total time in moderate to very active activity at the end of the day.

For an example, see page 45.

Example

_____
(day & date)

Time	Place	Food or Beverage	Amount
7:30 am	kitchen counter	orange juice	6 oz.
		bran flakes	1 cup
		w/ fat-free milk	1/4 cup
10:15 am	desk at work	coffee	6 oz.
		w/ cream	1 Tbsp.
		muffin	1 med.
Etc.			

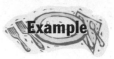

Food Group & No. of Servings	Social Situation	Hunger Level	Comments
Fruit (1)	ate alone	2	rushed, almost skipped it
Bread (1)			
Milk (1/4)			
none	sipped coffee and	1	morning pick-me-up habit
none	ate while I worked		
Bread (1)			

Example

Your Daily Pyramid Check-Up

For each food group, write the number of servings (whole or partial) you consumed today.

Fats, Oils & Sweets

Milk, Yogurt & Cheese 3

Meat, Poultry, Fish, Dry Beans, Eggs & Nuts 2

Vegetables 2

Fruits 2

Breads, Cereals, Rice & Pasta 5

Today did you consume...

	yes	no
enough servings to match your goal from the...		
Bread Group?	☐	☑
Vegetable Group?	☐	☑
Fruit Group?	☑	☐
Milk Group?	☑	☐
Meat Group?	☑	☐
Fats, Oils, and Sweets—from the Pyramid tip—*sparingly?*	☑	☐
mostly foods low in fat, saturated fat, and cholesterol?	☑	☐
a vitamin C-rich fruit or vegetable?	☑	☐
a vitamin A-rich fruit or vegetable?	☐	☑
3 servings of whole-grain foods?	☑	☐
8 or more cups of fluids?	☐	☑

Refer to page 16 for your personal Pyramid.
Refer to pages 187 and 188 for good sources of vitamins A and C.
Refer to page 184 for the fat content of foods.

Example

Your Physical Activity Record

Time of Day	Type of Physical Activity	Intensity	Time Spent
7:00 am	rode stationary bike while reading morning newspaper	3	10 minutes
5:15 pm	brisk walk to bus stop	3	10 minutes
7:30 pm	Jumped rope with the kids	4	5 minutes

Total time spent 25 minutes

Today, did you get at least 30 minutes
of moderate physical activity? . . . . yes ☐ no ☑

Example
45

Day One

_____
(day & date)

Time	Place	Food or Beverage	Amount

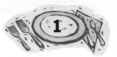

Food Group & No. of Servings	Social Situation	Hunger Level	Comments
_____	_____	_____	_____
_____	_____	_____	_____
_____	_____	_____	_____
_____	_____	_____	_____
_____	_____	_____	_____
_____	_____	_____	_____
_____	_____	_____	_____
_____	_____	_____	_____
_____	_____	_____	_____
_____	_____	_____	_____
_____	_____	_____	_____
_____	_____	_____	_____
_____	_____	_____	_____
_____	_____	_____	_____
_____	_____	_____	_____
_____	_____	_____	_____
_____	_____	_____	_____
_____	_____	_____	_____
_____	_____	_____	_____

Grate Ways with Veggies: Add grated or shredded vegetables—such as zucchini, spinach, or carrots—to lasagna, meat loaf, mashed potatoes, and other mixed meat, poultry, pasta, and other grain dishes.

Day One

47

Your Daily Pyramid Check-Up

For each food group, write the number of servings (whole or partial) you consumed today.

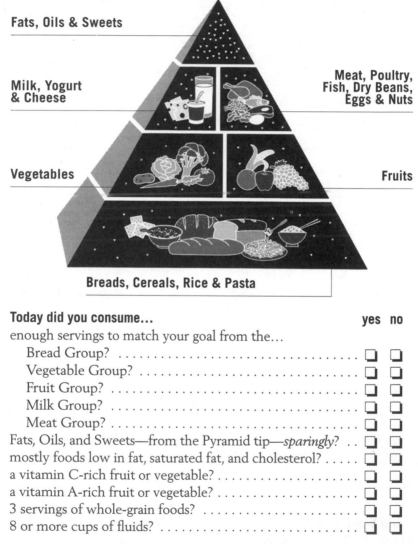

Fats, Oils & Sweets

Milk, Yogurt & Cheese

Meat, Poultry, Fish, Dry Beans, Eggs & Nuts

Vegetables

Fruits

Breads, Cereals, Rice & Pasta

Today did you consume...	yes	no
enough servings to match your goal from the...		
Bread Group?	❑	❑
Vegetable Group?	❑	❑
Fruit Group?	❑	❑
Milk Group?	❑	❑
Meat Group?	❑	❑
Fats, Oils, and Sweets—from the Pyramid tip—*sparingly?* ..	❑	❑
mostly foods low in fat, saturated fat, and cholesterol?	❑	❑
a vitamin C-rich fruit or vegetable?	❑	❑
a vitamin A-rich fruit or vegetable?	❑	❑
3 servings of whole-grain foods?	❑	❑
8 or more cups of fluids?	❑	❑

Refer to page 16 for your personal Pyramid.
Refer to pages 187 and 188 for good sources of vitamins A and C.
Refer to page 184 for the fat content of foods.

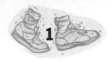

Your Physical Activity Record

Time of Day	Type of Physical Activity	Intensity	Time Spent

Total time spent _____

Today, did you get at least 30 minutes
of moderate physical activity? . . . . yes ☐ no ☐

An Active Mind-Set: Think physical activity! Look for
every chance to bend, reach, stretch, or move. Being in
that mind-set helps make physical activity a habit.

Day One

Day Two

_____
(day & date)

Time	Place	Food or Beverage	Amount

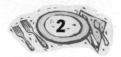

Food Group & No. of Servings	Social Situation	Hunger Level	Comments

Give It a High Five: Strive for five-a-day servings of fruits and vegetables—new types and all-time favorites. Try to eat a least one vitamin A-rich and one vitamin C-rich and one high-fiber choice daily.

Your Daily Pyramid Check-Up

For each food group, write the number of servings (whole or partial) you consumed today.

Fats, Oils & Sweets

Milk, Yogurt & Cheese

Meat, Poultry, Fish, Dry Beans, Eggs & Nuts

Vegetables

Fruits

Breads, Cereals, Rice & Pasta

Today did you consume...

enough servings to match your goal from the...

	yes	no
Bread Group?	☐	☐
Vegetable Group?	☐	☐
Fruit Group?	☐	☐
Milk Group?	☐	☐
Meat Group?	☐	☐
Fats, Oils, and Sweets—from the Pyramid tip—*sparingly*?	☐	☐
mostly foods low in fat, saturated fat, and cholesterol?	☐	☐
a vitamin C-rich fruit or vegetable?	☐	☐
a vitamin A-rich fruit or vegetable?	☐	☐
3 servings of whole-grain foods?	☐	☐
8 or more cups of fluids?	☐	☐

Refer to page 16 for your personal Pyramid.
Refer to pages 187 and 188 for good sources of vitamins A and C.
Refer to page 184 for the fat content of foods.

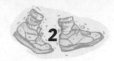

Your Physical Activity Record

Time of Day	Type of Physical Activity	Intensity	Time Spent

Total time spent _____

Today, did you get at least 30 minutes
of moderate physical activity? . . . . **yes☐ no☐**

Walk Your Talk: If you spend a lot of leisure time on
the phone, buy a portable one. Then walk—inside or
outdoors—as you chat with friends and family.

Day Two

Day Three

_____
(day & date)

Time	Place	Food or Beverage	Amount

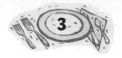

Food Group & No. of Servings	Social Situation	Hunger Level	Comments

New-Trition: Add variety, nutrients, and interest to your plate with new-to-you foods. When you shop, tuck an unfamiliar food into your cart. And when you eat out, order an appetizer portion of something new.

Day Three

Your Daily Pyramid Check-Up

For each food group, write the number of servings (whole or partial) you consumed today.

Fats, Oils & Sweets

Milk, Yogurt & Cheese

Meat, Poultry, Fish, Dry Beans, Eggs & Nuts

Vegetables

Fruits

Breads, Cereals, Rice & Pasta

Today did you consume...   yes   no

enough servings to match your goal from the...

Bread Group? .... ☐ ☐
Vegetable Group? .... ☐ ☐
Fruit Group? .... ☐ ☐
Milk Group? .... ☐ ☐
Meat Group? .... ☐ ☐
Fats, Oils, and Sweets—from the Pyramid tip—*sparingly?* .. ☐ ☐
mostly foods low in fat, saturated fat, and cholesterol? ..... ☐ ☐
a vitamin C-rich fruit or vegetable? .... ☐ ☐
a vitamin A-rich fruit or vegetable? .... ☐ ☐
3 servings of whole-grain foods? .... ☐ ☐
8 or more cups of fluids? .... ☐ ☐

Refer to page 16 for your personal Pyramid.
Refer to pages 187 and 188 for good sources of vitamins A and C.
Refer to page 184 for the fat content of foods.

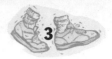

Your Physical Activity Record

Time of Day	Type of Physical Activity	Intensity	Time Spent
_____	_____	_____	_____
_____	_____	_____	_____
_____	_____	_____	_____
_____	_____	_____	_____
_____	_____	_____	_____
_____	_____	_____	_____
_____	_____	_____	_____
_____	_____	_____	_____
_____	_____	_____	_____
_____	_____	_____	_____
_____	_____	_____	_____
_____	_____	_____	_____
_____	_____	_____	_____
_____	_____	_____	_____
_____	_____	_____	_____
_____	_____	_____	_____

Total time spent _____

Today, did you get at least 30 minutes
of moderate physical activity? . . . . **yes☐ no☐**

The Housework Bonus: Sweep the sidewalk. Wash windows or the car. Vacuum your carpet. Many chores count toward the recommended 30 minutes of moderate physical activity daily.

Day Three

Day Four

(day & date)

Time	Place	Food or Beverage	Amount

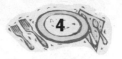

Food Group & No. of Servings	Social Situation	Hunger Level	Comments

Paint Your Plate: Color your plate healthy with all kinds of green, yellow, orange, and red vegetables and fruits. Many of these colorful foods are rich sources of beta carotene (vitamin A).

Day Four

Your Daily Pyramid Check-Up

For each food group, write the number of servings (whole or partial) you consumed today.

Fats, Oils & Sweets

Milk, Yogurt & Cheese

Meat, Poultry, Fish, Dry Beans, Eggs & Nuts

Vegetables

Fruits

Breads, Cereals, Rice & Pasta

Today did you consume...	yes	no
enough servings to match your goal from the...		
Bread Group?	☐	☐
Vegetable Group?	☐	☐
Fruit Group?	☐	☐
Milk Group?	☐	☐
Meat Group?	☐	☐
Fats, Oils, and Sweets—from the Pyramid tip—*sparingly*?	☐	☐
mostly foods low in fat, saturated fat, and cholesterol?	☐	☐
a vitamin C-rich fruit or vegetable?	☐	☐
a vitamin A-rich fruit or vegetable?	☐	☐
3 servings of whole-grain foods?	☐	☐
8 or more cups of fluids?	☐	☐

Refer to page 16 for your personal Pyramid.
Refer to pages 187 and 188 for good sources of vitamins A and C.
Refer to page 184 for the fat content of foods.

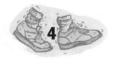
Your Physical Activity Record

Time of Day	Type of Physical Activity	Intensity	Time Spent

Total time spent _____

Today, did you get at least 30 minutes
    of moderate physical activity? . . . . **yes ☐ no ☐**

Rise and Shine: Wake up 30 minutes earlier. Start each
day with a brisk walk. Need encouragement? Schedule
walks with a neighbor.

Your Daily Pyramid Check-Up

For each food group, write the number of servings (whole or partial) you consumed today.

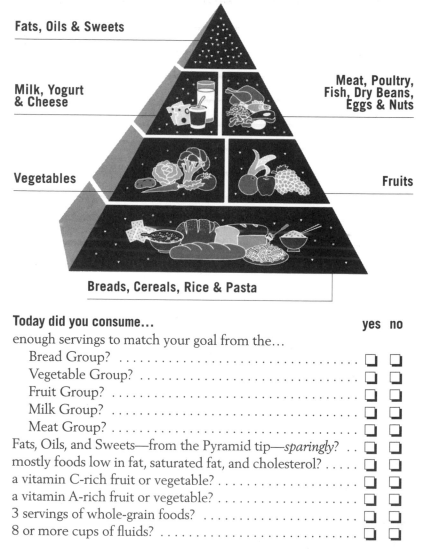

Fats, Oils & Sweets

Milk, Yogurt & Cheese

Meat, Poultry, Fish, Dry Beans, Eggs & Nuts

Vegetables

Fruits

Breads, Cereals, Rice & Pasta

Today did you consume...   yes   no

enough servings to match your goal from the...

Bread Group? . . . . ❏ ❏

Vegetable Group? . . . . ❏ ❏

Fruit Group? . . . . ❏ ❏

Milk Group? . . . . ❏ ❏

Meat Group? . . . . ❏ ❏

Fats, Oils, and Sweets—from the Pyramid tip—*sparingly?* . . ❏ ❏

mostly foods low in fat, saturated fat, and cholesterol? . . . . . ❏ ❏

a vitamin C-rich fruit or vegetable? . . . . ❏ ❏

a vitamin A-rich fruit or vegetable? . . . . ❏ ❏

3 servings of whole-grain foods? . . . . ❏ ❏

8 or more cups of fluids? . . . . ❏ ❏

Refer to page 16 for your personal Pyramid.
Refer to pages 187 and 188 for good sources of vitamins A and C.
Refer to page 184 for the fat content of foods.

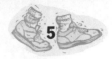

Your Physical Activity Record

Time of Day	Type of Physical Activity	Intensity	Time Spent

Total time spent _____

Today, did you get at least 30 minutes
of moderate physical activity? . . . . **yes ☐ no ☐**

Moves for Travelers: Pack comfortable clothes (or a
bathing suit) and footwear. If you bring your gear—jump
rope, walking shoes, or dumbbells to fill with water—you don't
need special facilities.

Day Six

_____
(day & date)

Time	Place	Food or Beverage	Amount

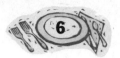

Food Group & No. of Servings	Social Situation	Hunger Level	Comments

Here's the Rub: Season meat, poultry, and fish with your favorite "rub"—such as grated citrus peel, garlic, and pepper, or an herb rub with marjoram, thyme, and basil. These rubs are sodium-free.

Day Six

67

Your Daily Pyramid Check-Up

For each food group, write the number of servings (whole or partial) you consumed today.

Fats, Oils & Sweets

Milk, Yogurt & Cheese

Meat, Poultry, Fish, Dry Beans, Eggs & Nuts

Vegetables

Fruits

Breads, Cereals, Rice & Pasta

Today did you consume...	yes	no
enough servings to match your goal from the...		
Bread Group?	❑	❑
Vegetable Group?	❑	❑
Fruit Group?	❑	❑
Milk Group?	❑	❑
Meat Group?	❑	❑
Fats, Oils, and Sweets—from the Pyramid tip—*sparingly*?	❑	❑
mostly foods low in fat, saturated fat, and cholesterol?	❑	❑
a vitamin C-rich fruit or vegetable?	❑	❑
a vitamin A-rich fruit or vegetable?	❑	❑
3 servings of whole-grain foods?	❑	❑
8 or more cups of fluids?	❑	❑

Refer to page 16 for your personal Pyramid.
Refer to pages 187 and 188 for good sources of vitamins A and C.
Refer to page 184 for the fat content of foods.

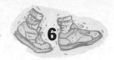

6

Your Physical Activity Record

Time of Day	Type of Physical Activity	Intensity	Time Spent
_____	_____	_____	_____
_____	_____	_____	_____
_____	_____	_____	_____
_____	_____	_____	_____
_____	_____	_____	_____
_____	_____	_____	_____
_____	_____	_____	_____
_____	_____	_____	_____
_____	_____	_____	_____
_____	_____	_____	_____
_____	_____	_____	_____
_____	_____	_____	_____
_____	_____	_____	_____
_____	_____	_____	_____
_____	_____	_____	_____
_____	_____	_____	_____
_____	_____	_____	_____
_____	_____	_____	_____

Total time spent _____

Today, did you get at least 30 minutes
of moderate physical activity? . . . . **yes** ☐ **no** ☐

Two-Step to Fitness: Dance as a leisure-time activity:
line dancing, disco dancing, salsa or ballroom dancing,
square dancing, or folk dancing. Even a moderate two-step
is good exercise.

Day Six

69

Day Seven

_____
(day & date)

Time	Place	Food or Beverage	Amount

Food Group & No. of Servings	Social Situation	Hunger Level	Comments

Insider Trading. Balance food choices during the day. Enjoy foods with less fat, then "spend" some savings on a higher-fat food, maybe ice cream. When you trade off fat, you trade off calories, too!

Your Daily Pyramid Check-Up

For each food group, write the number of servings (whole or partial) you consumed today.

Fats, Oils & Sweets

Milk, Yogurt & Cheese

Meat, Poultry, Fish, Dry Beans, Eggs & Nuts

Vegetables

Fruits

Breads, Cereals, Rice & Pasta

Today did you consume...	yes	no
enough servings to match your goal from the...		
Bread Group?	❏	❏
Vegetable Group?	❏	❏
Fruit Group?	❏	❏
Milk Group?	❏	❏
Meat Group?	❏	❏
Fats, Oils, and Sweets—from the Pyramid tip—*sparingly?*	❏	❏
mostly foods low in fat, saturated fat, and cholesterol?	❏	❏
a vitamin C-rich fruit or vegetable?	❏	❏
a vitamin A-rich fruit or vegetable?	❏	❏
3 servings of whole-grain foods?	❏	❏
8 or more cups of fluids?	❏	❏

Refer to page 16 for your personal Pyramid.
Refer to pages 187 and 188 for good sources of vitamins A and C.
Refer to page 184 for the fat content of foods.

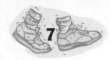

Your Physical Activity Record

Time of Day	Type of Physical Activity	Intensity	Time Spent

Total time spent _____

Today, did you get at least 30 minutes
of moderate physical activity? . . . . **yes ☐ no ☐**

Fitness Tid-Byte: For every hour you log on to the
computer, give yourself a five-minute (or longer)
physical activity break. Besides avoiding "computer potato"
syndrome, you'll relieve eyestrain.

Day Seven

Week One Check-Up

How many days this week did you...

	6-7	4-5	2-3	0-1
Consume at least 6 servings of breads, cereal, rice, pasta, and other grains?	❑	❑	❑	❑
Eat at least 3 whole-grain products?	❑	❑	❑	❑
Eat at least 3 servings of vegetables?	❑	❑	❑	❑
Eat at least 2 servings of fruits?	❑	❑	❑	❑
Consume enough calcium-rich dairy foods (at least 2 servings)?*	❑	❑	❑	❑
Eat protein-rich foods (meat, poultry, fish, beans, eggs, nuts) that add up to 5 to 7 ounces?	❑	❑	❑	❑
Go easy on foods that deliver energy, or calories, but few nutrients (fats and sweets)?	❑	❑	❑	❑
Drink at least 8 cups of fluids?	❑	❑	❑	❑
Meet your personal Pyramid goals?	❑	❑	❑	❑
Get at least 30 minutes of moderate activity?	❑	❑	❑	❑
Subtotal	___	___	___	___
	4 pts each	3 pts each	2 pts each	1 pt each

* More if you're a teen through age 24.
Pregnancy and breast-feeding require more, too.

Total Score ___

If you scored:

36-40: Great job! Now keep it up.

26-35: You're on roll in the right direction. Decide your next steps.

16-25: You've got the idea. And you have more stepping to do.

10-15: You've got a way to go—remember, even small changes make a difference.

Now look back at your goals and action plans for the week. Refer to page 36 and 37.

Success! Write this week's successes for healthier living.

___

___

___

___

Your Just Rewards. Celebrate success. Give yourself a personal (nonfood) reward.

_____

_____

_____

Something to Work On. Looking at this week, jot areas you could improve.

_____

_____

_____

Next Week, Next Steps. _As you start Week Two..._ Keeping this day-by-day diary is your first step toward a healthier life. If you've already made progress, keep it up! And if you need to adjust your action plan for the month, now's the time to do so. Remember, slow, gradual change is often more successful!

Your personal goals...   **Action plans for next week...**

For healthful eating...

_____   _____

_____   _____

_____   _____

For physical activity...

_____   _____

_____   _____

_____   _____

The Big Picture: In your action plan for smart eating, remember...what you eat over several days is what really counts—not what you eat for a single meal, snack, or day. Take that into account as you track your steps to fitness.

Your Weekly Check-Up

Day Eight

_____
(day & date)

Time	Place	Food or Beverage	Amount

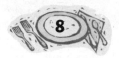

Food Group & No. of Servings	Social Situation	Hunger Level	Comments
_____	_____	_____	_____
_____	_____	_____	_____
_____	_____	_____	_____
_____	_____	_____	_____
_____	_____	_____	_____
_____	_____	_____	_____
_____	_____	_____	_____
_____	_____	_____	_____
_____	_____	_____	_____
_____	_____	_____	_____
_____	_____	_____	_____
_____	_____	_____	_____
_____	_____	_____	_____
_____	_____	_____	_____
_____	_____	_____	_____
_____	_____	_____	_____
_____	_____	_____	_____
_____	_____	_____	_____

Give Yourself a Break: Take time for lunch, even when you're under work pressure. With a break and a meal, you may avoid a dip in your afternoon energy level. And you just may be more productive!

Your Daily Pyramid Check-Up

For each food group, write the number of servings (whole or partial) you consumed today.

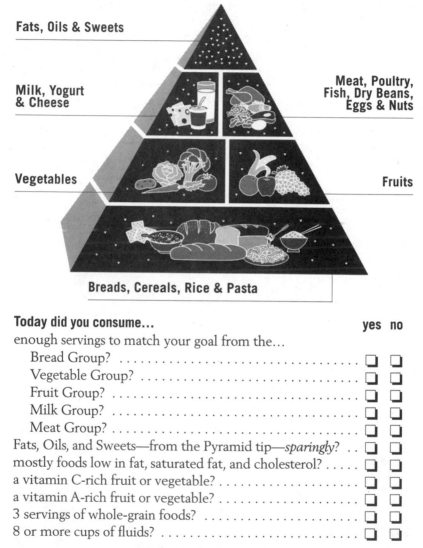

Fats, Oils & Sweets

Milk, Yogurt & Cheese

Meat, Poultry, Fish, Dry Beans, Eggs & Nuts

Vegetables

Fruits

Breads, Cereals, Rice & Pasta

Today did you consume...   yes no

enough servings to match your goal from the...

Bread Group? . . . . ☐ ☐

Vegetable Group? . . . . ☐ ☐

Fruit Group? . . . . ☐ ☐

Milk Group? . . . . ☐ ☐

Meat Group? . . . . ☐ ☐

Fats, Oils, and Sweets—from the Pyramid tip—*sparingly*? . . ☐ ☐

mostly foods low in fat, saturated fat, and cholesterol? . . . . . ☐ ☐

a vitamin C-rich fruit or vegetable? . . . . ☐ ☐

a vitamin A-rich fruit or vegetable? . . . . ☐ ☐

3 servings of whole-grain foods? . . . . ☐ ☐

8 or more cups of fluids? . . . . ☐ ☐

Refer to page 16 for your personal Pyramid.
Refer to pages 187 and 188 for good sources of vitamins A and C.
Refer to page 184 for the fat content of foods.

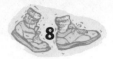

Your Physical Activity Record

Time of Day	Type of Physical Activity	Intensity	Time Spent

Total time spent _____

Today, did you get at least 30 minutes
of moderate physical activity? . . . . **yes ☐ no ☐**

Going Solo: At home or as you travel, walk safely alone
in shopping malls and museums. Try power walking—
pump your arms for a better workout. Wear comfortable
walking shoes!

Day Eight

Day Nine

_____
(day & date)

Time	Place	Food or Beverage	Amount

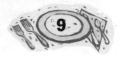

Food Group & No. of Servings	Social Situation	Hunger Level	Comments

Go Skinless: Today's advice: before or after cooking poultry, remove the skin—and cut the fat content in half! Cooking with the skin on keeps poultry moist.

Day Nine

Your Daily Pyramid Check-Up

For each food group, write the number of servings (whole or partial) you consumed today.

Fats, Oils & Sweets

Milk, Yogurt & Cheese

Meat, Poultry, Fish, Dry Beans, Eggs & Nuts

Vegetables

Fruits

Breads, Cereals, Rice & Pasta

Today did you consume...	yes	no
enough servings to match your goal from the...		
Bread Group?	☐	☐
Vegetable Group?	☐	☐
Fruit Group?	☐	☐
Milk Group?	☐	☐
Meat Group?	☐	☐
Fats, Oils, and Sweets—from the Pyramid tip—*sparingly*?	☐	☐
mostly foods low in fat, saturated fat, and cholesterol?	☐	☐
a vitamin C-rich fruit or vegetable?	☐	☐
a vitamin A-rich fruit or vegetable?	☐	☐
3 servings of whole-grain foods?	☐	☐
8 or more cups of fluids?	☐	☐

Refer to page 16 for your personal Pyramid.
Refer to pages 187 and 188 for good sources of vitamins A and C.
Refer to page 184 for the fat content of foods.

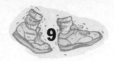

Your Physical Activity Record

Time of Day	Type of Physical Activity	Intensity	Time Spent

Total time spent _____

Today, did you get at least 30 minutes
of moderate physical activity? . . . . **yes ☐ no ☐**

Video Workouts: Next time you rent a movie, rent an
exercise video, too. Work out with the video—before
or after the movie, or as a brief intermission.

Day Nine

Day Ten

_____
(day & date)

Time	Place	Food or Beverage	Amount

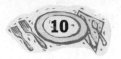

Food Group & No. of Servings	Social Situation	Hunger Level	Comments

Snack Smart: Rather than think of snacks as extras, choose those that contribute food-group servings—fruits, vegetables, grains, and calcium-rich dairy foods—to your personal Pyramid.

Your Daily Pyramid Check-Up

For each food group, write the number of servings (whole or partial) you consumed today.

Fats, Oils & Sweets

Milk, Yogurt & Cheese

Meat, Poultry, Fish, Dry Beans, Eggs & Nuts

Vegetables

Fruits

Breads, Cereals, Rice & Pasta

Today did you consume...

enough servings to match your goal from the...

	yes	no
Bread Group?	☐	☐
Vegetable Group?	☐	☐
Fruit Group?	☐	☐
Milk Group?	☐	☐
Meat Group?	☐	☐
Fats, Oils, and Sweets—from the Pyramid tip—*sparingly?*	☐	☐
mostly foods low in fat, saturated fat, and cholesterol?	☐	☐
a vitamin C-rich fruit or vegetable?	☐	☐
a vitamin A-rich fruit or vegetable?	☐	☐
3 servings of whole-grain foods?	☐	☐
8 or more cups of fluids?	☐	☐

Refer to page 16 for your personal Pyramid.
Refer to pages 187 and 188 for good sources of vitamins A and C.
Refer to page 184 for the fat content of foods.

Monthly Nutrition Companion

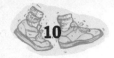

Your Physical Activity Record

Time of Day	Type of Physical Activity	Intensity	Time Spent

Total time spent _____

Today, did you get at least 30 minutes
of moderate physical activity? . . . . **yes ☐ no ☐**

One-Minute Moves: At your desk waiting for a
phone call or on-line computer connection? Do some
deep knee bends, toe touches, stretches, or isometric exercises.

Day Eleven

_____
(day & date)

Time	Place	Food or Beverage	Amount

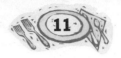

Food Group & No. of Servings	Social Situation	Hunger Level	Comments

Take a Fruit to Lunch: Tuck an apple, tangerine, two plums or kiwis, grapes, cherries, dried fruits, or other fruit into your briefcase, tote, or lunch bag. They're a low-fat and tasty snack choice!

Day Eleven

Your Daily Pyramid Check-Up

For each food group, write the number of servings (whole or partial) you consumed today.

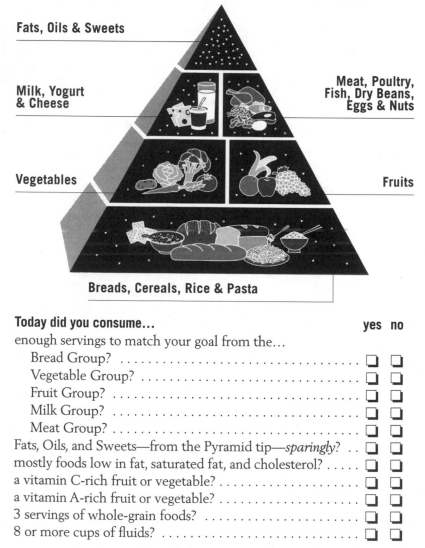

Fats, Oils & Sweets

Milk, Yogurt & Cheese

Meat, Poultry, Fish, Dry Beans, Eggs & Nuts

Vegetables

Fruits

Breads, Cereals, Rice & Pasta

Today did you consume...	yes	no
enough servings to match your goal from the...		
Bread Group?	❑	❑
Vegetable Group?	❑	❑
Fruit Group?	❑	❑
Milk Group?	❑	❑
Meat Group?	❑	❑
Fats, Oils, and Sweets—from the Pyramid tip—*sparingly*?	❑	❑
mostly foods low in fat, saturated fat, and cholesterol?	❑	❑
a vitamin C-rich fruit or vegetable?	❑	❑
a vitamin A-rich fruit or vegetable?	❑	❑
3 servings of whole-grain foods?	❑	❑
8 or more cups of fluids?	❑	❑

Refer to page 16 for your personal Pyramid.
Refer to pages 187 and 188 for good sources of vitamins A and C.
Refer to page 184 for the fat content of foods.

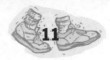

Your Physical Activity Record

Time of Day	Type of Physical Activity	Intensity	Time Spent
_____	_____	_____	_____
_____	_____	_____	_____
_____	_____	_____	_____
_____	_____	_____	_____
_____	_____	_____	_____
_____	_____	_____	_____
_____	_____	_____	_____
_____	_____	_____	_____
_____	_____	_____	_____
_____	_____	_____	_____
_____	_____	_____	_____
_____	_____	_____	_____
_____	_____	_____	_____
_____	_____	_____	_____
_____	_____	_____	_____
_____	_____	_____	_____
_____	_____	_____	_____

Total time spent _____

Today, did you get at least 30 minutes
of moderate physical activity? . . . . **yes ☐ no ☐**

Quality Time: Play actively with your kids, grandkids,
or pets. A game of Frisbee, tag, or catch can be fun for
everyone—even the dog! If you have snow, make a
snowman.

Day Eleven

Day Twelve

_____

Time	Place	Food or Beverage	Amount

Monthly Nutrition Companion

Food Group & No. of Servings	Social Situation	Hunger Level	Comments

Dressed for Success: Go easy on regular salad dressings. Just two tablespoons add about 150 calories to an otherwise low-calorie salad. Try a splash of flavored vinegar or a low-calorie or fat-free variety.

Your Daily Pyramid Check-Up

For each food group, write the number of servings (whole or partial) you consumed today.

Fats, Oils & Sweets

Milk, Yogurt & Cheese

Meat, Poultry, Fish, Dry Beans, Eggs & Nuts

Vegetables

Fruits

Breads, Cereals, Rice & Pasta

Today did you consume...	yes	no
enough servings to match your goal from the...		
Bread Group?	☐	☐
Vegetable Group?	☐	☐
Fruit Group?	☐	☐
Milk Group?	☐	☐
Meat Group?	☐	☐
Fats, Oils, and Sweets—from the Pyramid tip—*sparingly*?	☐	☐
mostly foods low in fat, saturated fat, and cholesterol?	☐	☐
a vitamin C-rich fruit or vegetable?	☐	☐
a vitamin A-rich fruit or vegetable?	☐	☐
3 servings of whole-grain foods?	☐	☐
8 or more cups of fluids?	☐	☐

Refer to page 16 for your personal Pyramid.
Refer to pages 187 and 188 for good sources of vitamins A and C.
Refer to page 184 for the fat content of foods.

Your Physical Activity Record

Time of Day	Type of Physical Activity	Intensity	Time Spent

Total time spent _____

Today, did you get at least 30 minutes
of moderate physical activity? . . . . **yes ☐ no ☐**

Adventure Travel: Plan active family trips or weekend outings—go canoeing, hiking, or skiing. If you prefer to "beach it," make long beach walks part of your recreation.

Day Twelve

Day Thirteen

_____

(day & date)

Time	Place	Food or Beverage	Amount

Food Group & No. of Servings	Social Situation	Hunger Level	Comments

Lean Your Cuisine: Use mostly cooking methods that add little or no fat. Broil or grill, roast, braise, stew, steam, poach, stir-fry, or microwave foods, rather than fry them.

Your Daily Pyramid Check-Up

For each food group, write the number of servings (whole or partial) you consumed today.

Fats, Oils & Sweets

Milk, Yogurt & Cheese

Meat, Poultry, Fish, Dry Beans, Eggs & Nuts

Vegetables

Fruits

Breads, Cereals, Rice & Pasta

Today did you consume...	yes	no
enough servings to match your goal from the...		
Bread Group?	☐	☐
Vegetable Group?	☐	☐
Fruit Group?	☐	☐
Milk Group?	☐	☐
Meat Group?	☐	☐
Fats, Oils, and Sweets—from the Pyramid tip—*sparingly*?	☐	☐
mostly foods low in fat, saturated fat, and cholesterol?	☐	☐
a vitamin C-rich fruit or vegetable?	☐	☐
a vitamin A-rich fruit or vegetable?	☐	☐
3 servings of whole-grain foods?	☐	☐
8 or more cups of fluids?	☐	☐

Refer to page 16 for your personal Pyramid.
Refer to pages 187 and 188 for good sources of vitamins A and C.
Refer to page 184 for the fat content of foods.

Your Physical Activity Record

Time of Day	Type of Physical Activity	Intensity	Time Spent

Total time spent _____

Today, did you get at least 30 minutes
of moderate physical activity? . . . . **yes**☐ **no**☐

Your Personal Gym: Do you own exercise equipment?
Make time to use it! Use your exercise bike, treadmill, or
rowing machine while you catch up on the day's TV news.

Day Thirteen

Day Fourteen

_____
(day & date)

Time	Place	Food or Beverage	Amount

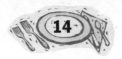

Food Group & No. of Servings	Social Situation	Hunger Level	Comments

Nature's Fast Food: For quick, easy snacks, keep your refrigerator stocked with raw vegetables and fruits. If you're a "big dipper," have a nutritious, low-fat dip —low-fat cottage cheese puréed with herbs.

Your Daily Pyramid Check-Up

For each food group, write the number of servings (whole or partial) you consumed today.

Fats, Oils & Sweets

Milk, Yogurt & Cheese

Meat, Poultry, Fish, Dry Beans, Eggs & Nuts

Vegetables

Fruits

Breads, Cereals, Rice & Pasta

Today did you consume...	yes	no
enough servings to match your goal from the...		
Bread Group?	❏	❏
Vegetable Group?	❏	❏
Fruit Group?	❏	❏
Milk Group?	❏	❏
Meat Group?	❏	❏
Fats, Oils, and Sweets—from the Pyramid tip—*sparingly?*	❏	❏
mostly foods low in fat, saturated fat, and cholesterol?	❏	❏
a vitamin C-rich fruit or vegetable?	❏	❏
a vitamin A-rich fruit or vegetable?	❏	❏
3 servings of whole-grain foods?	❏	❏
8 or more cups of fluids?	❏	❏

Refer to page 16 for your personal Pyramid.
Refer to pages 187 and 188 for good sources of vitamins A and C.
Refer to page 184 for the fat content of foods.

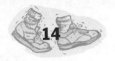
Your Physical Activity Record

Time of Day	Type of Physical Activity	Intensity	Time Spent

Total time spent _____

Today, did you get at least 30 minutes
of moderate physical activity? . . . . **yes** ☐ **no** ☐

Pedal Power: Put your car keys away. Use your bike
for short errands. (For safety, wear your helmet.) Ride
your bike to work or a nearby friend's home. No bike?
Then walk if you can.

Day Fourteen

Week Two Check-Up

How many days this week did you...	6-7	4-5	2-3	0-1
Consume at least 6 servings of breads, cereal, rice, pasta, and other grains?	❏	❏	❏	❏
Eat at least 3 whole-grain products?	❏	❏	❏	❏
Eat at least 3 servings of vegetables?	❏	❏	❏	❏
Eat at least 2 servings of fruits?	❏	❏	❏	❏
Consume enough calcium-rich dairy foods (at least 2 servings)?*	❏	❏	❏	❏
Eat protein-rich foods (meat, poultry, fish, beans, eggs, nuts) that add up to 5 to 7 ounces?	❏	❏	❏	❏
Go easy on foods that deliver energy, or calories, but few nutrients (fats and sweets)? .	❏	❏	❏	❏
Drink at least 8 cups of fluids?	❏	❏	❏	❏
Meet your personal Pyramid goals?	❏	❏	❏	❏
Get at least 30 minutes of moderate activity? .	❏	❏	❏	❏

* More if you're a teen through age 24.
Pregnancy and breast-feeding require more, too.

Subtotal ___ ___ ___ ___

4 pts each   3 pts each   2 pts each   1 pt each

Total Score ___

If you scored:

36-40: Great job! Now keep it up.

26-35: You're on roll in the right direction. Decide your next steps.

16-25: You've got the idea. And you have more stepping to do.

10-15: You've got a way to go—remember, even small changes make a difference.

Now look back at your goals and action plans for the week. Refer to page 75.

Success! Write this week's successes for healthier living.

_____

_____

_____

_____

Your Just Rewards. Celebrate success. Give yourself a personal (nonfood) reward.

_____

_____

Something to Work On. Looking at this week, jot areas you could improve.

_____

_____

_____

Next Week, Next Steps. *As you start Week Three...* This is the mid-point in your month's action plan. Are you sticking with your strategies for fitness? If you need to get back on track, this is the time to do so.

Your personal goals...   **Action plans for next week...**

For healthful eating...

_____

_____

_____

For physical activity...

_____

_____

The Yo-Yo Problem! For a trimmer shape, avoid the cycle of losing and regaining. A yo-yo dieter needs fewer and fewer calories to maintain weight, making weight loss harder and harder. A long-term action plan—with gradual, permanent changes in your eating and activity level—is the effective and healthy way to keep trim.

Day Fifteen

_____
(day & date)

Time	Place	Food or Beverage	Amount

15

Food Group & No. of Servings	Social Situation	Hunger Level	Comments

Perfect Pairings: Enhance iron absorption from grain products and legumes. Pair them with vitamin C-rich fruits. Top oatmeal with berries, or drink orange juice with a peanut butter sandwich.

Day Fifteen

107

Your Daily Pyramid Check-Up

For each food group, write the number of servings (whole or partial) you consumed today.

Fats, Oils & Sweets

Milk, Yogurt & Cheese

Meat, Poultry, Fish, Dry Beans, Eggs & Nuts

Vegetables

Fruits

Breads, Cereals, Rice & Pasta

Today did you consume...	**yes**	**no**
enough servings to match your goal from the...		
Bread Group?	❑	❑
Vegetable Group?	❑	❑
Fruit Group?	❑	❑
Milk Group?	❑	❑
Meat Group?	❑	❑
Fats, Oils, and Sweets—from the Pyramid tip—*sparingly*? . .	❑	❑
mostly foods low in fat, saturated fat, and cholesterol?	❑	❑
a vitamin C-rich fruit or vegetable?	❑	❑
a vitamin A-rich fruit or vegetable?	❑	❑
3 servings of whole-grain foods?	❑	❑
8 or more cups of fluids?	❑	❑

Refer to page 16 for your personal Pyramid.
Refer to pages 187 and 188 for good sources of vitamins A and C.
Refer to page 184 for the fat content of foods.

Your Physical Activity Record

Time of Day	Type of Physical Activity	Intensity	Time Spent
_____	_____	_____	_____
_____	_____	_____	_____
_____	_____	_____	_____
_____	_____	_____	_____
_____	_____	_____	_____
_____	_____	_____	_____
_____	_____	_____	_____
_____	_____	_____	_____
_____	_____	_____	_____
_____	_____	_____	_____
_____	_____	_____	_____
_____	_____	_____	_____
_____	_____	_____	_____
_____	_____	_____	_____
_____	_____	_____	_____
_____	_____	_____	_____
_____	_____	_____	_____

Total time spent _____

Today, did you get at least 30 minutes
  of moderate physical activity? . . . . **yes**☐ **no**☐

Tune It Up: Short on time? Just turn up the music on
your CD or tape player—and dance! Like walking and
running, dancing is a weight-bearing activity that's good for
your bones.

Day Sixteen

_____
(day & date)

Time	Place	Food or Beverage	Amount

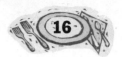

Food Group & No. of Servings	Social Situation	Hunger Level	Comments

Incredible Edibles: When you think nutrition, think taste. And when you think taste, think nutrition. The pleasure of eating and good health go hand in hand!

Day Sixteen

Your Daily Pyramid Check-Up

For each food group, write the number of servings (whole or partial) you consumed today.

Fats, Oils & Sweets

Milk, Yogurt & Cheese

Meat, Poultry, Fish, Dry Beans, Eggs & Nuts

Vegetables

Fruits

Breads, Cereals, Rice & Pasta

Today did you consume...   yes no
enough servings to match your goal from the...

Bread Group? . . . . ❑ ❑
Vegetable Group? . . . . ❑ ❑
Fruit Group? . . . . ❑ ❑
Milk Group? . . . . ❑ ❑
Meat Group? . . . . ❑ ❑
Fats, Oils, and Sweets—from the Pyramid tip—*sparingly?* . . ❑ ❑
mostly foods low in fat, saturated fat, and cholesterol? . . . . . ❑ ❑
a vitamin C-rich fruit or vegetable? . . . . ❑ ❑
a vitamin A-rich fruit or vegetable? . . . . ❑ ❑
3 servings of whole-grain foods? . . . . ❑ ❑
8 or more cups of fluids? . . . . ❑ ❑

Refer to page 16 for your personal Pyramid.
Refer to pages 187 and 188 for good sources of vitamins A and C.
Refer to page 184 for the fat content of foods.

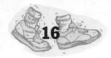

Your Physical Activity Record

Time of Day	Type of Physical Activity	Intensity	Time Spent

Total time spent _____

Today, did you get at least 30 minutes
of moderate physical activity? . . . . **yes ☐ no ☐**

Stair-Stepping: Take stairs instead of the elevator or
escalator. Walking up stairs is a great heart exerciser
and calorie burner!

Day Sixteen

16

Day Seventeen

_____
(day & date)

Time	Place	Food or Beverage	Amount

Food Group & No. of Servings	Social Situation	Hunger Level	Comments

The Great Divide: For meal variety divide your plate in pie-shaped sections. Fill 75 percent of the plate with grain products, vegetables, and fruits—the rest with meat, poultry, or fish. Serve milk, too!

Day Seventeen

Your Daily Pyramid Check-Up

For each food group, write the number of servings (whole or partial) you consumed today.

Fats, Oils & Sweets

Milk, Yogurt & Cheese

Meat, Poultry, Fish, Dry Beans, Eggs & Nuts

Vegetables

Fruits

Breads, Cereals, Rice & Pasta

Today did you consume...

enough servings to match your goal from the...

	yes	no
Bread Group?	❏	❏
Vegetable Group?	❏	❏
Fruit Group?	❏	❏
Milk Group?	❏	❏
Meat Group?	❏	❏
Fats, Oils, and Sweets—from the Pyramid tip—*sparingly?*	❏	❏
mostly foods low in fat, saturated fat, and cholesterol?	❏	❏
a vitamin C-rich fruit or vegetable?	❏	❏
a vitamin A-rich fruit or vegetable?	❏	❏
3 servings of whole-grain foods?	❏	❏
8 or more cups of fluids?	❏	❏

Refer to page 16 for your personal Pyramid.
Refer to pages 187 and 188 for good sources of vitamins A and C.
Refer to page 184 for the fat content of foods.

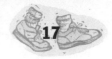

Your Physical Activity Record

Time of Day	Type of Physical Activity	Intensity	Time Spent

Total time spent _____

Today, did you get at least 30 minutes
of moderate physical activity? . . . . **yes ☐ no ☐**

Personal "Power Assist": Push your lawn mower
instead of using the power-assisted drive. Or if you're fit,
shovel snow by hand, and give the snowblower a rest.

Day Seventeen

Day Eighteen

_____
(day & date)

Time	Place	Food or Beverage	Amount

Food Group & No. of Servings	Social Situation	Hunger Level	Comments

Bone Up: Fortify lasagna, meat loaf, mashed potatoes, and soups with dry milk, evaporated skim milk, or plain yogurt. Sprinkle cheese on potatoes, vegetables, soups, and salads. Calcium's a bone builder!

Day Eighteen

Your Daily Pyramid Check-Up

For each food group, write the number of servings (whole or partial) you consumed today.

Fats, Oils & Sweets

Milk, Yogurt & Cheese

Meat, Poultry, Fish, Dry Beans, Eggs & Nuts

Vegetables

Fruits

Breads, Cereals, Rice & Pasta

Today did you consume...   yes no

enough servings to match your goal from the...

Bread Group? . . . . ❑ ❑

Vegetable Group? . . . . ❑ ❑

Fruit Group? . . . . ❑ ❑

Milk Group? . . . . ❑ ❑

Meat Group? . . . . ❑ ❑

Fats, Oils, and Sweets—from the Pyramid tip—*sparingly?* . . ❑ ❑

mostly foods low in fat, saturated fat, and cholesterol? . . . . . ❑ ❑

a vitamin C-rich fruit or vegetable? . . . . ❑ ❑

a vitamin A-rich fruit or vegetable? . . . . ❑ ❑

3 servings of whole-grain foods? . . . . ❑ ❑

8 or more cups of fluids? . . . . ❑ ❑

Refer to page 16 for your personal Pyramid.
Refer to pages 187 and 188 for good sources of vitamins A and C.
Refer to page 184 for the fat content of foods.

Your Physical Activity Record

Time of Day	Type of Physical Activity	Intensity	Time Spent

Total time spent _____

Today, did you get at least 30 minutes
of moderate physical activity? . . . . **yes ☐ no☐**

Far Out: Park at the far end of the parking lot for a
longer walk. Get off the bus a stop ahead. Then walk the
rest of the way to your destination.

Day Eighteen

Day Nineteen

_____

Time	Place	Food or Beverage	Amount
_____	_____	_____	_____
_____	_____	_____	_____
_____	_____	_____	_____
_____	_____	_____	_____
_____	_____	_____	_____
_____	_____	_____	_____
_____	_____	_____	_____
_____	_____	_____	_____
_____	_____	_____	_____
_____	_____	_____	_____
_____	_____	_____	_____
_____	_____	_____	_____
_____	_____	_____	_____
_____	_____	_____	_____
_____	_____	_____	_____
_____	_____	_____	_____
_____	_____	_____	_____
_____	_____	_____	_____
_____	_____	_____	_____

Food Group & No. of Servings	Social Situation	Hunger Level	Comments

Well Equipped: Buy a fat-separating pitcher. Use it to degrease gravy, drippings, and broth. The position of the spout lets you pour out the flavorful liquid from the bottom and leave the fat behind.

Day Nineteen

Your Daily Pyramid Check-Up

For each food group, write the number of servings (whole or partial) you consumed today.

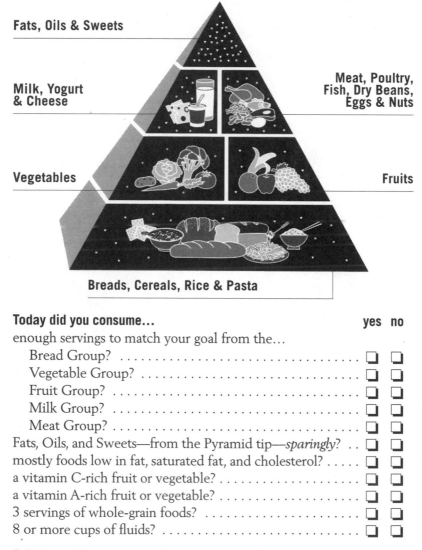

Fats, Oils & Sweets

Milk, Yogurt & Cheese

Meat, Poultry, Fish, Dry Beans, Eggs & Nuts

Vegetables

Fruits

Breads, Cereals, Rice & Pasta

Today did you consume...   yes   no

enough servings to match your goal from the...
	yes	no
Bread Group?	☐	☐
Vegetable Group?	☐	☐
Fruit Group?	☐	☐
Milk Group?	☐	☐
Meat Group?	☐	☐
Fats, Oils, and Sweets—from the Pyramid tip—*sparingly*?	☐	☐
mostly foods low in fat, saturated fat, and cholesterol?	☐	☐
a vitamin C-rich fruit or vegetable?	☐	☐
a vitamin A-rich fruit or vegetable?	☐	☐
3 servings of whole-grain foods?	☐	☐
8 or more cups of fluids?	☐	☐

Refer to page 16 for your personal Pyramid.
Refer to pages 187 and 188 for good sources of vitamins A and C.
Refer to page 184 for the fat content of foods.

Your Physical Activity Record

Time of Day	Type of Physical Activity	Intensity	Time Spent

Total time spent _____

Today, did you get at least 30 minutes
of moderate physical activity? . . . . **yes ☐ no ☐**

Walk Together, Talk Together: Before or after dinner,
walk with your family. It's a great time for talking
together, too! If you have an infant, use a baby carrier
rather than a stroller.

Day Nineteen

Day Twenty

_____
(day & date)

Time	Place	Food or Beverage	Amount

Food Group & No. of Servings	Social Situation	Hunger Level	Comments

Label-Able: A food labeled "low-fat" may not have fewer calories. Even if it does, remember, eating two or three times more of a low-fat food may not offer any calorie savings!

Your Daily Pyramid Check-Up

For each food group, write the number of servings (whole or partial) you consumed today.

Fats, Oils & Sweets

Milk, Yogurt & Cheese

Meat, Poultry, Fish, Dry Beans, Eggs & Nuts

Vegetables

Fruits

Breads, Cereals, Rice & Pasta

Today did you consume...	yes	no
enough servings to match your goal from the...		
Bread Group?	☐	☐
Vegetable Group?	☐	☐
Fruit Group?	☐	☐
Milk Group?	☐	☐
Meat Group?	☐	☐
Fats, Oils, and Sweets—from the Pyramid tip—*sparingly?*	☐	☐
mostly foods low in fat, saturated fat, and cholesterol?	☐	☐
a vitamin C-rich fruit or vegetable?	☐	☐
a vitamin A-rich fruit or vegetable?	☐	☐
3 servings of whole-grain foods?	☐	☐
8 or more cups of fluids?	☐	☐

Refer to page 16 for your personal Pyramid.
Refer to pages 187 and 188 for good sources of vitamins A and C.
Refer to page 184 for the fat content of foods.

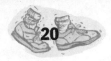

Your Physical Activity Record

Time of Day	Type of Physical Activity	Intensity	Time Spent
_____	_____	_____	_____
_____	_____	_____	_____
_____	_____	_____	_____
_____	_____	_____	_____
_____	_____	_____	_____
_____	_____	_____	_____
_____	_____	_____	_____
_____	_____	_____	_____
_____	_____	_____	_____
_____	_____	_____	_____
_____	_____	_____	_____
_____	_____	_____	_____
_____	_____	_____	_____
_____	_____	_____	_____
_____	_____	_____	_____
_____	_____	_____	_____
_____	_____	_____	_____
_____	_____	_____	_____

Total time spent _____

Today, did you get at least 30 minutes
of moderate physical activity? . . . . **yes** ☐ **no** ☐

For the Hobbyist: Take up an active hobby: perhaps
furniture refinishing, gardening, bicycling, bread baking
(knead by hand), tennis, or home remodeling.

Day Twenty

Day Twenty-One

_____
(day & date)

Time	Place	Food or Beverage	Amount

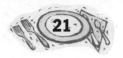

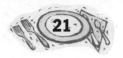

21

Food Group & No. of Servings	Social Situation	Hunger Level	Comments

Milk It—For All It's Worth: During your coffee break, reach for milk. No place to buy it? Bring some from home and keep it in the office fridge. Or order caffe latte or cappuccino, both made with steamed milk.

Day Twenty-One

131

Your Daily Pyramid Check-Up

For each food group, write the number of servings (whole or partial) you consumed today.

Fats, Oils & Sweets

Milk, Yogurt & Cheese

Meat, Poultry, Fish, Dry Beans, Eggs & Nuts

Vegetables

Fruits

Breads, Cereals, Rice & Pasta

Today did you consume...	yes	no
enough servings to match your goal from the...		
Bread Group?	☐	☐
Vegetable Group?	☐	☐
Fruit Group?	☐	☐
Milk Group?	☐	☐
Meat Group?	☐	☐
Fats, Oils, and Sweets—from the Pyramid tip—*sparingly*?	☐	☐
mostly foods low in fat, saturated fat, and cholesterol?	☐	☐
a vitamin C-rich fruit or vegetable?	☐	☐
a vitamin A-rich fruit or vegetable?	☐	☐
3 servings of whole-grain foods?	☐	☐
8 or more cups of fluids?	☐	☐

Refer to page 16 for your personal Pyramid.
Refer to pages 187 and 188 for good sources of vitamins A and C.
Refer to page 184 for the fat content of foods.

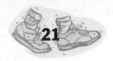

Your Physical Activity Record

Time of Day	Type of Physical Activity	Intensity	Time Spent

Total time spent _____

Today, did you get at least 30 minutes
of moderate physical activity? . . . . **yes ☐ no ☐**

Break the Habit: During your lunch hour or coffee break, make a habit of walking around the building—inside or outdoors. You'll burn energy rather than be tempted to snack.

Day Twenty-One

133

Week Three Check-Up

How many days this week did you...	6-7	4-5	2-3	0-1
Consume at least 6 servings of breads, cereal, rice, pasta, and other grains?	❑	❑	❑	❑
Eat at least 3 whole-grain products?	❑	❑	❑	❑
Eat at least 3 servings of vegetables?	❑	❑	❑	❑
Eat at least 2 servings of fruits?	❑	❑	❑	❑
Consume enough calcium-rich dairy foods (at least 2 servings)?*	❑	❑	❑	❑
Eat protein-rich foods (meat, poultry, fish, beans, eggs, nuts) that add up to 5 to 7 ounces?	❑	❑	❑	❑
Go easy on foods that deliver energy, or calories, but few nutrients (fats and sweets)?	❑	❑	❑	❑
Drink at least 8 cups of fluids?	❑	❑	❑	❑
Meet your personal Pyramid goals?	❑	❑	❑	❑
Get at least 30 minutes of moderate activity?	❑	❑	❑	❑

* More if you're a teen through age 24.
Pregnancy and breast-feeding require more, too.

Subtotal ___ ___ ___ ___

4 pts each   3 pts each   2 pts each   1 pt each

Total Score ____

If you scored:

36-40: Great job! Now keep it up.

26-35: You're on roll in the right direction. Decide your next steps.

16-25: You've got the idea. And you have more stepping to do.

10-15: You've got a way to go—remember, even small changes make a difference.

Now look back at your goals and action plans for the week. Refer to page 105.

Success! Write this week's successes for healthier living.

_____

_____

_____

_____

Your Just Rewards. Celebrate success. Give yourself a personal (nonfood) reward.

_____

_____

_____

Something to Work On. Looking at this week, jot areas you could improve.

_____

_____

_____

Next Week, Next Steps. *As you start Week Four...* You're nearing the home stretch for this month. Check your overall goals and strategies again. Make some adjustments if you need to. And keep on going so that you can finish the month with success!

Your personal goals...   **Action plans for next week...**

For healthful eating...

_____   _____

_____   _____

_____   _____

For physical activity...

_____   _____

_____   _____

_____   _____

Lean Advantage. If you step up to a physically active lifestyle, you'll gradually build more lean muscle. Muscle uses more energy than body fat. So if you're lean, you may be able to consume more calories without gaining weight!

Day Twenty-Two

(day & date)

Time	Place	Food or Beverage	Amount

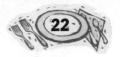

Food Group & No. of Servings	Social Situation	Hunger Level	Comments

Fish-y Story: Look for water-packed canned tuna, salmon, and other fish. Besides the milder flavor, they have significantly less fat. Canned salmon and sardines with edible bones supply calcium, too.

Day Twenty-Two

137

Your Daily Pyramid Check-Up

For each food group, write the number of servings (whole or partial) you consumed today.

Fats, Oils & Sweets

Milk, Yogurt & Cheese

Meat, Poultry, Fish, Dry Beans, Eggs & Nuts

Vegetables

Fruits

Breads, Cereals, Rice & Pasta

Today did you consume...	yes	no
enough servings to match your goal from the...		
Bread Group?	❏	❏
Vegetable Group?	❏	❏
Fruit Group?	❏	❏
Milk Group?	❏	❏
Meat Group?	❏	❏
Fats, Oils, and Sweets—from the Pyramid tip—*sparingly?*	❏	❏
mostly foods low in fat, saturated fat, and cholesterol?	❏	❏
a vitamin C-rich fruit or vegetable?	❏	❏
a vitamin A-rich fruit or vegetable?	❏	❏
3 servings of whole-grain foods?	❏	❏
8 or more cups of fluids?	❏	❏

Refer to page 16 for your personal Pyramid.
Refer to pages 187 and 188 for good sources of vitamins A and C.
Refer to page 184 for the fat content of foods.

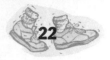

22

Your Physical Activity Record

Time of Day	Type of Physical Activity	Intensity	Time Spent
_____	_____	_____	_____
_____	_____	_____	_____
_____	_____	_____	_____
_____	_____	_____	_____
_____	_____	_____	_____
_____	_____	_____	_____
_____	_____	_____	_____
_____	_____	_____	_____
_____	_____	_____	_____
_____	_____	_____	_____
_____	_____	_____	_____
_____	_____	_____	_____
_____	_____	_____	_____
_____	_____	_____	_____
_____	_____	_____	_____
_____	_____	_____	_____
_____	_____	_____	_____
_____	_____	_____	_____

Total time spent _____

Today, did you get at least 30 minutes
    of moderate physical activity? . . . . yes ☐ no ☐

Splish-Splash: Skip the drive-through car wash. Wash
the car yourself. Giving your pet a bath may give you a
real workout, too!

Day Twenty-Two

Day Twenty-Three

_____
(day & date)

Time	Place	Food or Beverage	Amount

Food Group & No. of Servings	Social Situation	Hunger Level	Comments

Saucy Up: Purée fruit or cooked vegetables for poultry, fish, meat, and rice or pasta dishes. Perhaps glaze poultry with puréed berries or peaches or toss pasta with an herbed broccoli purée.

Your Daily Pyramid Check-Up

For each food group, write the number of servings (whole or partial) you consumed today.

Fats, Oils & Sweets

Milk, Yogurt & Cheese

Meat, Poultry, Fish, Dry Beans, Eggs & Nuts

Vegetables

Fruits

Breads, Cereals, Rice & Pasta

Today did you consume...

enough servings to match your goal from the...

	yes	no
Bread Group?	☐	☐
Vegetable Group?	☐	☐
Fruit Group?	☐	☐
Milk Group?	☐	☐
Meat Group?	☐	☐
Fats, Oils, and Sweets—from the Pyramid tip—*sparingly?*	☐	☐
mostly foods low in fat, saturated fat, and cholesterol?	☐	☐
a vitamin C-rich fruit or vegetable?	☐	☐
a vitamin A-rich fruit or vegetable?	☐	☐
3 servings of whole-grain foods?	☐	☐
8 or more cups of fluids?	☐	☐

Refer to page 16 for your personal Pyramid.
Refer to pages 187 and 188 for good sources of vitamins A and C.
Refer to page 184 for the fat content of foods.

Your Physical Activity Record

Time of Day	Type of Physical Activity	Intensity	Time Spent
_____	_____	_____	_____
_____	_____	_____	_____
_____	_____	_____	_____
_____	_____	_____	_____
_____	_____	_____	_____
_____	_____	_____	_____
_____	_____	_____	_____
_____	_____	_____	_____
_____	_____	_____	_____
_____	_____	_____	_____
_____	_____	_____	_____
_____	_____	_____	_____
_____	_____	_____	_____
_____	_____	_____	_____
_____	_____	_____	_____
_____	_____	_____	_____
_____	_____	_____	_____

Total time spent _____

Today, did you get at least 30 minutes
of moderate physical activity? . . . . yes☐ no☐

Family Affair: Learn a new activity that your whole
family can enjoy together: perhaps ice skating, in-line
skating, or tennis. Remember the knee pads and helmet
if you take up in-line skating.

Day Twenty-Three

Day Twenty-Four

_____
(day & date)

Time	Place	Food or Beverage	Amount

Food Group & No. of Servings	Social Situation	Hunger Level	Comments

Menu Language: Be aware of menu terms that may mean more fat—au gratin, batter fried, bearnaise, breaded, creamed, double crust, en croute, french fried, pastry, sautéed, scalloped, and with gravy.

Day Twenty-Four

145

Your Daily Pyramid Check-Up

For each food group, write the number of servings (whole or partial) you consumed today.

Fats, Oils & Sweets

Milk, Yogurt & Cheese

Meat, Poultry, Fish, Dry Beans, Eggs & Nuts

Vegetables

Fruits

Breads, Cereals, Rice & Pasta

Today did you consume...

	yes	no
enough servings to match your goal from the...		
Bread Group?	❏	❏
Vegetable Group?	❏	❏
Fruit Group?	❏	❏
Milk Group?	❏	❏
Meat Group?	❏	❏
Fats, Oils, and Sweets—from the Pyramid tip—*sparingly*?	❏	❏
mostly foods low in fat, saturated fat, and cholesterol?	❏	❏
a vitamin C-rich fruit or vegetable?	❏	❏
a vitamin A-rich fruit or vegetable?	❏	❏
3 servings of whole-grain foods?	❏	❏
8 or more cups of fluids?	❏	❏

Refer to page 16 for your personal Pyramid.
Refer to pages 187 and 188 for good sources of vitamins A and C.
Refer to page 184 for the fat content of foods.

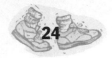

Your Physical Activity Record

Time of Day	Type of Physical Activity	Intensity	Time Spent
_____	_____	_____	_____
_____	_____	_____	_____
_____	_____	_____	_____
_____	_____	_____	_____
_____	_____	_____	_____
_____	_____	_____	_____
_____	_____	_____	_____
_____	_____	_____	_____
_____	_____	_____	_____
_____	_____	_____	_____
_____	_____	_____	_____
_____	_____	_____	_____
_____	_____	_____	_____
_____	_____	_____	_____
_____	_____	_____	_____

Total time spent _____

Today, did you get at least 30 minutes
   of moderate physical activity? . . . . **yes ☐ no ☐**

Class Act: Sign up for an adult-ed class at your
community school: perhaps volleyball, racquetball,
fencing, or tap dancing.

Day Twenty-Four

Day Twenty-Five

_____
(day & date)

Time	Place	Food or Beverage	Amount

Food Group & No. of Servings	Social Situation	Hunger Level	Comments

Size Wise: Whether it's a sandwich, fries, or other fast food item, "big," "deluxe," and "super" portions mean more calories, and more fat, cholesterol, and sodium. The regular size may be enough!

Your Daily Pyramid Check-Up

For each food group, write the number of servings (whole or partial) you consumed today.

Fats, Oils & Sweets

Milk, Yogurt & Cheese

Meat, Poultry, Fish, Dry Beans, Eggs & Nuts

Vegetables

Fruits

Breads, Cereals, Rice & Pasta

Today did you consume...

	yes	no
enough servings to match your goal from the...		
Bread Group?	☐	☐
Vegetable Group?	☐	☐
Fruit Group?	☐	☐
Milk Group?	☐	☐
Meat Group?	☐	☐
Fats, Oils, and Sweets—from the Pyramid tip—*sparingly*?	☐	☐
mostly foods low in fat, saturated fat, and cholesterol?	☐	☐
a vitamin C-rich fruit or vegetable?	☐	☐
a vitamin A-rich fruit or vegetable?	☐	☐
3 servings of whole-grain foods?	☐	☐
8 or more cups of fluids?	☐	☐

Refer to page 16 for your personal Pyramid.
Refer to pages 187 and 188 for good sources of vitamins A and C.
Refer to page 184 for the fat content of foods.

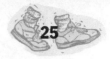

Your Physical Activity Record

Time of Day	Type of Physical Activity	Intensity	Time Spent
_____	_____	_____	_____
_____	_____	_____	_____
_____	_____	_____	_____
_____	_____	_____	_____
_____	_____	_____	_____
_____	_____	_____	_____
_____	_____	_____	_____
_____	_____	_____	_____
_____	_____	_____	_____
_____	_____	_____	_____
_____	_____	_____	_____
_____	_____	_____	_____
_____	_____	_____	_____
_____	_____	_____	_____
_____	_____	_____	_____
_____	_____	_____	_____
_____	_____	_____	_____
_____	_____	_____	_____

Total time spent _____

Today, did you get at least 30 minutes
of moderate physical activity? . . . . **yes**☐ **no**☐

Pet-Agree: Get a dog and walk together. No dog?
Then walk your cat on a leash.

Day Twenty-Five

Day Twenty-Six

_____

(day & date)

Time	Place	Food or Beverage	Amount

Food Group & No. of Servings	Social Situation	Hunger Level	Comments

The Whole Story: For your 3 daily whole-grain foods try, whole-grain breads and mixed stir-fries, soups, and salads, made with barley, brown rice, buckwheat, bulgur, millet, quinoa, or rye or wheat berries.

Day Twenty-Six

Your Daily Pyramid Check-Up

For each food group, write the number of servings (whole or partial) you consumed today.

Fats, Oils & Sweets

Milk, Yogurt & Cheese

Meat, Poultry, Fish, Dry Beans, Eggs & Nuts

Vegetables

Fruits

Breads, Cereals, Rice & Pasta

Today did you consume...	yes	no
enough servings to match your goal from the...		
Bread Group?	❑	❑
Vegetable Group?	❑	❑
Fruit Group?	❑	❑
Milk Group?	❑	❑
Meat Group?	❑	❑
Fats, Oils, and Sweets—from the Pyramid tip—*sparingly?* . .	❑	❑
mostly foods low in fat, saturated fat, and cholesterol?	❑	❑
a vitamin C-rich fruit or vegetable?	❑	❑
a vitamin A-rich fruit or vegetable?	❑	❑
3 servings of whole-grain foods?	❑	❑
8 or more cups of fluids?	❑	❑

Refer to page 16 for your personal Pyramid.
Refer to pages 187 and 188 for good sources of vitamins A and C.
Refer to page 184 for the fat content of foods.

Your Physical Activity Record

Time of Day	Type of Physical Activity	Intensity	Time Spent

Total time spent _____

Today, did you get at least 30 minutes
of moderate physical activity? . . . . **yes☐ no☐**

On the Road? On a long drive, take regular breaks.
You and your passengers—including pets—will ride more
comfortably and stay alert after a brisk walk or other physical
activity.

Day Twenty-Six
155

Day Twenty-Seven

_____
(day & date)

Time	Place	Food or Beverage	Amount

Food Group & No. of Servings	Social Situation	Hunger Level	Comments

Get the Skinny on Meat. Choose lean cuts: round and loin cuts of beef, and loin and leg cuts of pork and lamb. Look for ground beef labeled "95 percent lean," and deli meats labeled "low-fat" or "lean."

Day Twenty-Seven

Your Daily Pyramid Check-Up

For each food group, write the number of servings (whole or partial) you consumed today.

Fats, Oils & Sweets

Milk, Yogurt & Cheese

Meat, Poultry, Fish, Dry Beans, Eggs & Nuts

Vegetables

Fruits

Breads, Cereals, Rice & Pasta

Today did you consume...	yes	no
enough servings to match your goal from the...		
Bread Group?	❏	❏
Vegetable Group?	❏	❏
Fruit Group?	❏	❏
Milk Group?	❏	❏
Meat Group?	❏	❏
Fats, Oils, and Sweets—from the Pyramid tip—*sparingly*?	❏	❏
mostly foods low in fat, saturated fat, and cholesterol?	❏	❏
a vitamin C-rich fruit or vegetable?	❏	❏
a vitamin A-rich fruit or vegetable?	❏	❏
3 servings of whole-grain foods?	❏	❏
8 or more cups of fluids?	❏	❏

Refer to page 16 for your personal Pyramid.
Refer to pages 187 and 188 for good sources of vitamins A and C.
Refer to page 184 for the fat content of foods.

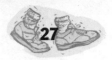
Your Physical Activity Record

Time of Day	Type of Physical Activity	Intensity	Time Spent

Total time spent _____

Today, did you get at least 30 minutes
of moderate physical activity? . . . . **yes☐ no☐**

Check Your TV Guide: Look for a televised workout or
yoga class to set you in motion.

Day Twenty-Seven

159

Day Twenty-Eight

_____
(day & date)

Time	Place	Food or Beverage	Amount

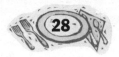

Food Group & No. of Servings	Social Situation	Hunger Level	Comments

Pack and Go: "Chill out" with an insulated container full of nutrition: raw veggies and fresh fruit; sandwiches with whole-grain bread, lean meat, cheese, and veggies; low-fat yogurt; boxed juice and milk.

Day Twenty-Eight

Your Daily Pyramid Check-Up

For each food group, write the number of servings (whole or partial) you consumed today.

Fats, Oils & Sweets

Milk, Yogurt & Cheese

Meat, Poultry, Fish, Dry Beans, Eggs & Nuts

Vegetables

Fruits

Breads, Cereals, Rice & Pasta

Today did you consume...

enough servings to match your goal from the...

	yes	no
Bread Group?	❏	❏
Vegetable Group?	❏	❏
Fruit Group?	❏	❏
Milk Group?	❏	❏
Meat Group?	❏	❏
Fats, Oils, and Sweets—from the Pyramid tip—*sparingly?*	❏	❏
mostly foods low in fat, saturated fat, and cholesterol?	❏	❏
a vitamin C-rich fruit or vegetable?	❏	❏
a vitamin A-rich fruit or vegetable?	❏	❏
3 servings of whole-grain foods?	❏	❏
8 or more cups of fluids?	❏	❏

Refer to page 16 for your personal Pyramid.
Refer to pages 187 and 188 for good sources of vitamins A and C.
Refer to page 184 for the fat content of foods.

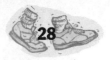

Your Physical Activity Record

Time of Day	Type of Physical Activity	Intensity	Time Spent

Total time spent _____

Today, did you get at least 30 minutes
of moderate physical activity? . . . . **yes ☐ no ☐**

On the Far Side: Use the restroom, drinking fountain,
or pay phone that's at the other end of the building.
You'll get a longer walk.

Day Twenty-Eight

Week Four Check-Up

How many days this week did you...	6-7	4-5	2-3	0-1
Consume at least 6 servings of breads, cereal, rice, pasta, and other grains?	❑	❑	❑	❑
Eat at least 3 whole-grain products?	❑	❑	❑	❑
Eat at least 3 servings of vegetables?	❑	❑	❑	❑
Eat at least 2 servings of fruits?	❑	❑	❑	❑
Consume enough calcium-rich dairy foods (at least 2 servings)?*	❑	❑	❑	❑
Eat protein-rich foods (meat, poultry, fish, beans, eggs, nuts) that add up to 5 to 7 ounces?	❑	❑	❑	❑
Go easy on foods that deliver energy, or calories, but few nutrients (fats and sweets)?	❑	❑	❑	❑
Drink at least 8 cups of fluids?	❑	❑	❑	❑
Meet your personal Pyramid goals?	❑	❑	❑	❑
Get at least 30 minutes of moderate activity?	❑	❑	❑	❑
Subtotal	___	___	___	___
	4 pts each	3 pts each	2 pts each	1 pt each

* More if you're a teen through age 24.
Pregnancy and breast-feeding require more, too.

Total Score ____

If you scored:

36-40: Great job! Now keep it up.

26-35: You're on roll in the right direction. Decide your next steps.

16-25: You've got the idea. And you have more stepping to do.

10-15: You've got a way to go—remember, even small changes make a difference.

Now look back at your goals and action plans for the week. Refer to page 135.

Success! Write this week's successes for healthier living.

_____

_____

_____

_____

Your Just Rewards. Celebrate success. Give yourself a personal (nonfood) reward.

_____

_____

_____

Something to Work On. Looking at this week, jot areas you could improve.

_____

_____

_____

Next Week, Next Steps. *As you continue...* If you decide to make this a monthly rather than 4-week (28-day) planner, you have a few bonus days left! Use them to reinforce your goals, strategies, and successes.

Your personal goals...   **Action plans for next week...**

For healthful eating...

_____   _____

_____   _____

_____   _____

For physical activity...

_____   _____

_____   _____

_____   _____

Program Your PC. Use your PC—portion control—to moderate your fat intake. Extra large portions of higher-fat foods add up to extra large amounts of fat and calories, too. Take your portion size into account in your action plan for healthy eating!

Your Weekly Check-Up

Day Twenty-Nine

(day & date)

Time	Place	Food or Beverage	Amount

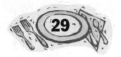

Food Group & No. of Servings	Social Situation	Hunger Level	Comments

Party Tid-Bite: Denying yourself holiday or party foods, or feeling guilty when you do enjoy them, doesn't fit in a healthy eating strategy—or a joyous occasion! Enjoy these special foods in small portions.

Day Twenty-Nine

Your Daily Pyramid Check-Up

For each food group, write the number of servings (whole or partial) you consumed today.

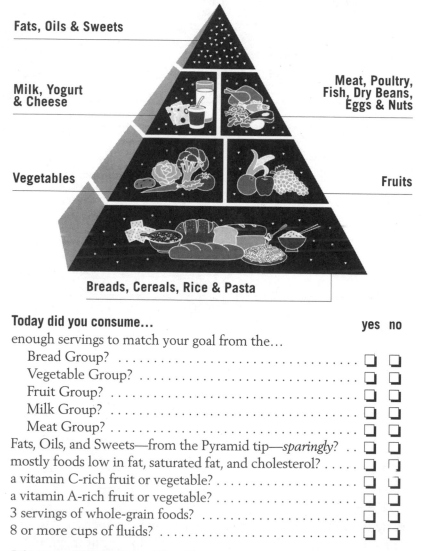

Fats, Oils & Sweets

Milk, Yogurt & Cheese

Meat, Poultry, Fish, Dry Beans, Eggs & Nuts

Vegetables

Fruits

Breads, Cereals, Rice & Pasta

Today did you consume...

enough servings to match your goal from the...

	yes	no
Bread Group?	☐	☐
Vegetable Group?	☐	☐
Fruit Group?	☐	☐
Milk Group?	☐	☐
Meat Group?	☐	☐
Fats, Oils, and Sweets—from the Pyramid tip—*sparingly?*	☐	☐
mostly foods low in fat, saturated fat, and cholesterol?	☐	☐
a vitamin C-rich fruit or vegetable?	☐	☐
a vitamin A-rich fruit or vegetable?	☐	☐
3 servings of whole-grain foods?	☐	☐
8 or more cups of fluids?	☐	☐

Refer to page 16 for your personal Pyramid.
Refer to pages 187 and 188 for good sources of vitamins A and C.
Refer to page 184 for the fat content of foods.

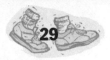

Your Physical Activity Record

Time of Day	Type of Physical Activity	Intensity	Time Spent
_____	_____	_____	_____
_____	_____	_____	_____
_____	_____	_____	_____
_____	_____	_____	_____
_____	_____	_____	_____
_____	_____	_____	_____
_____	_____	_____	_____
_____	_____	_____	_____
_____	_____	_____	_____
_____	_____	_____	_____
_____	_____	_____	_____
_____	_____	_____	_____
_____	_____	_____	_____
_____	_____	_____	_____
_____	_____	_____	_____
_____	_____	_____	_____
_____	_____	_____	_____
_____	_____	_____	_____

Total time spent _____

Today, did you get at least 30 minutes
   of moderate physical activity? . . . . **yes☐ no☐**

These Shoes Are Meant for Walkin': To make walking
more fun, change your route. Explore new places. Keeping
up an activity routine is easier if you include a fresh experience
from time to time!

Day Twenty-Nine

169

Day Thirty

(day & date)

Time	Place	Food or Beverage	Amount

Food Group & No. of Servings	Social Situation	Hunger Level	Comments

Gifts from Your Kitchen: A basket of fruit you picked; a "bean bag" of dry legumes with a chile or bean soup recipe; a raw veggie basket with a stir-fry herb blend; or fresh bread, baked in your bread machine.

Day Thirty

Your Daily Pyramid Check-Up

For each food group, write the number of servings (whole or partial) you consumed today.

Fats, Oils & Sweets

Milk, Yogurt & Cheese

Meat, Poultry, Fish, Dry Beans, Eggs & Nuts

Vegetables

Fruits

Breads, Cereals, Rice & Pasta

Today did you consume...	**yes**	**no**
enough servings to match your goal from the...		
Bread Group?	☐	☐
Vegetable Group?	☐	☐
Fruit Group?	☐	☐
Milk Group?	☐	☐
Meat Group?	☐	☐
Fats, Oils, and Sweets—from the Pyramid tip—*sparingly*?	☐	☐
mostly foods low in fat, saturated fat, and cholesterol?	☐	☐
a vitamin C-rich fruit or vegetable?	☐	☐
a vitamin A-rich fruit or vegetable?	☐	☐
3 servings of whole-grain foods?	☐	☐
8 or more cups of fluids?	☐	☐

Refer to page 16 for your personal Pyramid.
Refer to pages 187 and 188 for good sources of vitamins A and C.
Refer to page 184 for the fat content of foods.

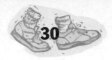

Your Physical Activity Record

Time of Day	Type of Physical Activity	Intensity	Time Spent

Total time spent _____

Today, did you get at least 30 minutes
   of moderate physical activity? . . . . **yes ☐ no ☐**

Cost-Conscious Fitness: To keep your arms strong, use canned foods from your kitchen shelves as weights. You can do 25 repetitions while you heat something in the microwave oven!

Day Thirty-One

_____
(day & date)

Time	Place	Food or Beverage	Amount

Food Group & No. of Servings	Social Situation	Hunger Level	Comments

Savor Ethnic Flavor: Middle Eastern hummus, Asian chicken satay, Italian polenta, Thai vegetable-noodle dishes, Brazilian black bean soup, Moroccan couscous, and Greek cucumber-yogurt dip.

Day Thirty-One

Your Daily Pyramid Check-Up

For each food group, write the number of servings (whole or partial) you consumed today.

Fats, Oils & Sweets

Milk, Yogurt & Cheese

Meat, Poultry, Fish, Dry Beans, Eggs & Nuts

Vegetables

Fruits

Breads, Cereals, Rice & Pasta

Today did you consume...	yes	no
enough servings to match your goal from the...		
Bread Group?	☐	☐
Vegetable Group?	☐	☐
Fruit Group?	☐	☐
Milk Group?	☐	☐
Meat Group?	☐	☐
Fats, Oils, and Sweets—from the Pyramid tip—*sparingly*?	☐	☐
mostly foods low in fat, saturated fat, and cholesterol?	☐	☐
a vitamin C-rich fruit or vegetable?	☐	☐
a vitamin A-rich fruit or vegetable?	☐	☐
3 servings of whole-grain foods?	☐	☐
8 or more cups of fluids?	☐	☐

Refer to page 16 for your personal Pyramid.
Refer to pages 187 and 188 for good sources of vitamins A and C.
Refer to page 184 for the fat content of foods.

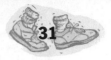

Your Physical Activity Record

Time of Day	Type of Physical Activity	Intensity	Time Spent

Total time spent _____

Today, did you get at least 30 minutes
of moderate physical activity? . . . . **yes ☐ no ☐**

Flying High. On a long plane trip, walk up and down
the aisle at least once an hour. Ask for an aisle seat so you
can easily get up and move. Do simple stretching exercises, too,
to avoid feeling stiff.

Day Thirty-One

Monthly Check-Up

Tracking your month's food choices and physical activities day-by-day has likely given you a closer look at your overall eating and activity patterns: what you choose, why, when, where, and how! If you've taken your action plans to heart, you've already "stepped toward fitness."

As you look back over the past month, you might complete the questionnaire "All About You..." on page 3 again. Then compare your answers now to what you said four weeks ago.

Jot down changes you made this month in your overall lifestyle—your eating and physical activity patterns—that are helping you achieve your fitness goals.

_____

_____

_____

_____

If you've accomplished any of your personal goals (for example, lost 2 pounds), record them!

_____

_____

_____

_____

If you've gone astray anywhere, record that, too… and how you could do better next month.

Problem areas...   **How you could do better...**

_____   _____

_____   _____

_____   _____

_____   _____

If you've kept with your plan, your month's small steps have already helped you make some big leaps toward fitness!

Looking Ahead: Your Next Steps Now, how can you maintain your new patterns—after all, your pay-off comes with a life-long commitment! And what new goals and action plans will you set for the weeks and month ahead?

Your personal goals...   **Your action plans...**

_____	_____
_____	_____
_____	_____
_____	_____
_____	_____
_____	_____
_____	_____
_____	_____
_____	_____
_____	_____
_____	_____
_____	_____

To put next month's plan into action—and to move closer to your fitness goals—continue to keep your day-by-day diary and evaluate your progress along the way. Start the month with another *Monthly Nutrition Companion!*

Sign On!

Make next month's goals and action plans part of your ongoing contract for fitness.

_____   _____
(your signature)   (date)

When You
Need to
Know More

AS YOU SET YOUR GOALS, choose your strategies, keep your record, and then evaluate your actions, you may need to know more about healthful eating. If so, turn to the next few pages.

About Some Nutrients in Food *183*
    Sorting the Fat, Saturated Fat, and
       Cholesterol, Too
    Vitamin A: Good Picks
    Vitamin C: Not Just From Citrus!
    Calcium: How Much in Food?
    Iron… From Many Sources
    Food's Fiber Factor
    Sodium: In Which Foods?

Healthy Weight—For You! *195*

In the Mood for Food!. *197*

How to Get Sound Advice About Healthful Eating *199*

When You Need to Know More

About Some Nutrients In Food

FOOD CONTAINS 40 OR SO NUTRIENTS, each with unique roles in promoting your health. Charts on the following pages show food sources of nutrients and food substances that are challenges for many people:

➤ fat, saturated fat, cholesterol, and sodium, commonly consumed in excess amounts;

➤ vitamins A and C, calcium, iron, and fiber, which often come up short.

Sorting the Fat, Saturated Fat, and Cholesterol, Too

Many of today's health problems are linked to a high-fat eating pattern. On average, Americans consume 34 percent of their energy, or calories, from fat.

Health experts advise less: no more than 30 percent of energy from fat, and no more than 10 percent from saturated fat. And limit cholesterol intake to 300 milligrams or less each day. Here's what that means at three calorie levels:

	CALORIES		
	1,600	2,200	2,800
Total fat (grams)	53	73	93
Saturated fat (grams)	17	24	31
Cholesterol (milligrams)	300	300	300

Fat and Cholesterol Finder

Fat comes from foods of plant and animal origin, but the amount varies. Most fruits and vegetables and many grain products are low in fat. And only animal products contain cholesterol.

Use the following chart to find amounts of fat, saturated fat, and cholesterol, in typical food choices. Nutrition Facts on food labels can help you learn more.

	Total fat (g)	Saturated fatty acids (g)	Cholesterol (mg)
Breads, Cereals, Rice, and Pasta			
Bread, 1 slice			
white	1	trace	trace
whole-wheat	1	trace	0
Bagel, with egg, 1	1	trace	14
Biscuit, 1 medium	3	1	2
Roll, dinner, 1	2	trace	0
Croissant, 1 medium	12	7	62
Muffin, 1 large	6	2	44
Pancake, 1 medium	3	1	26
Waffle, 1 medium	5	2	39
Doughnut, yeast, 1	14	5	21
Danish pastry, 1 (2 oz.)	13	4	49
Oatmeal, cooked, 1/2 cup	1	trace	0
Shredded wheat, 1 lg. biscuit	trace	trace	0
Granola, 1/3 cup	10	2	0
Rice, white, cooked, 1/2 cup	trace	trace	0
Fried rice (with egg 1/2 cup and vegetables),	6	1	21
Cookie, 1 medium			
Oatmeal	3	1	5
Chocolate chip	4	1	6
Cake, devil's-food, frosted, 1/12 of 8-inch	16	5	32
Vegetables			
Potatoes			
Boiled, 1/2 cup	trace	trace	0
Potato salad, 1/2 cup	8	1	50
French fries, 10 strips	8	3	0
Au gratin, 1/2 cup	9	4	19
Chips, 1 oz.	10	3	0
Cabbage, 1/2 cup			
Cooked	trace	trace	0
Creamy coleslaw	11	2	6

	Total fat (g)	Saturated fatty acids (g)	Cholesterol (mg)
Celery & carrot sticks, 8	trace	0	0
Stir-fried vegetables, 1/2 cup	trace	trace	0

Fruits

	Total fat (g)	Saturated fatty acids (g)	Cholesterol (mg)
Apple, 1 medium	trace	trace	0
Avocado, 1/2 medium	15	2	0
Banana, 1 medium	1	trace	0
Olives, 5 large			
Green	3	trace	0
Ripe	3	trace	0
Orange, 1 medium	trace	trace	0
Peach, 1 medium	trace	trace	0
Strawberries, 5 berries	1	trace	0
Mixed fruit cup with cream dressing, 1/2 cup	3	2	9

Milk, Yogurt, Cheese

	Total fat (g)	Saturated fatty acids (g)	Cholesterol (mg)
Milk, 1 cup			
Whole	8	5	33
2% reduced-fat	5	3	18
1% low-fat	3	2	10
Fat-free	trace	trace	4
Yogurt, 1 cup			
Nonfat, plain	trace	trace	4
Low-fat, plain	4	2	15
Low-fat, fruit flavored	3	2	10
Cottage cheese, 1/2 cup			
Creamed	5	3	16
Low-fat, 1% fat	1	1	5
Cheese, 1 oz.			
Natural cheddar	9	6	29
Mozzarella, part-skim	5	3	16
Process American	9	6	27
Vanilla ice cream, 1/2 cup	7	4	27
Vanilla ice milk, 1/2 cup	3	2	9
Frozen yogurt, 1/2 cup	2	1	8

Meats, Poultry, Fish, Beans, Eggs, and Nuts

	Total fat (g)	Saturated fatty acids (g)	Cholesterol (mg)
Beef			
Lean cut (eye of round), roasted, 3 oz.			
Lean and fat	11	4	61
Lean only	4	2	59
Fattier cut (chuck blade), braised, 3 oz.			
Lean and fat	22	9	88
Lean only	11	4	90

	Total fat (g)	Saturated fatty acids (g)	Cholesterol (mg)
Ground, cooked, 3 oz. patty			
Regular	17	7	76
Lean	16	6	73
Extra lean	14	5	71
Pork center loin, roasted, 3 oz.			
Lean and fat	11	4	68
Lean	8	3	67
Beef liver, braised, 3 oz.	4	2	331
Chicken, light and dark meat, roasted, 3 oz.			
With skin	12	3	74
Without skin	6	2	75
Halibut fillet, baked, 3 oz.	1	trace	49
Tuna, canned, 3 oz.			
In oil	7	1	25
In water	1	trace	25
Crabs, hardshell, steamed, 2 med.	2	trace	95
Shrimp, steamed or boiled, 8 extra large	2	trace	160
Frankfurters, 2 (3 oz.)	27	10	47
Legumes, cooked, 1/2 c.	trace	trace	0
Peanut butter, 2 Tbsp.	16	3	0
Sunflower seeds, 2 Tbsp.	10	1	0
Egg, large, cooked, 1			
Yolk	5	2	213
White	0	0	0

Fats, Oils, Sweets

	Total fat (g)	Saturated fatty acids (g)	Cholesterol (mg)
Butter, 1 Tbsp.	12	7	31
Butter-margarine blend, 1 Tbsp.	12	5	16
Margarine, 1 Tbsp.			
Soft	12	2	0
Stick	12	2	0
Liquid (squeezable)	12	2	0
Diet	6	1	0
Vegetable oil (corn), 1 Tbsp.	14	2	0
Hydrogenated vegetable shortening, 1 Tbsp.	13	3	0
Salad dressing, 1 Tbsp.			
Mayonnaise (regular)	12	2	7
Mayonnaise, reduced calorie	5	1	5
Mayonnaise-type	7	1	4
Mayonnaise-type, reduced calorie	4	1	4

	Total fat (g)	Saturated fatty acids (g)	Cholesterol (mg)
Italian	7	1	0
Italian, low-calorie	1	trace	1
Cream, 1 Tbsp.			
Sour	3	2	6
Light (table)	3	2	10
Nondairy, frozen	1	trace	0
Cream cheese, 1 Tbsp.	5	3	16
Pie, apple, 1/8 of 9-inch	22	5	0
Cheesecake, 1/12 of 9-inch	25	10	86
Sherbet, 1/2 cup	2	1	7
Milk chocolate bar, 1 oz.	9	5	6

Source: Human Nutrition Information Service/United States Department of Agriculture, "Choose a Diet Low in Fat, Saturated Fat, and Cholesterol," *Home and Garden Bulletin* Number 253-4, July, 1993.

Vitamin A: Good Picks

Food provides vitamin A in two ways: 1) as retinol in foods of animal origin, and 2) from carotenoids, such as beta carotene in fruits and vegetables, which changes to vitamin A in your body. Many dark green leafy, red, yellow, and orange fruits and vegetables contain carotenoids.

Starting at age 11, most males need about 1,000 retinol equivalents (RE) of vitamin A; females need about 800 REs. Both the retinol and beta carotene content of food determine the retinol equivalents. These foods are among the good sources:

Food	Vitamin A (RE)*
Beef liver, cooked (3 ounces)	9,085
Sweet potato, mashed (1/2 cup)	2,800
Carrot (1 medium)	2,025
Kale, boiled (1/2 cup)	480
Mango, medium (1/2)	405
Turnip greens, cooked (1/2 cup)	395
Spinach, raw (1 cup)	375
Papaya, medium (1/2)	305
Red bell pepper, raw (1/2 cup)	285
Apricot (3)	275
Cantaloupe (1/2 cup)	260
Milk, skim (1 cup)	150
Romaine lettuce (1 cup)	145
Egg, large (1)	95

Food	Vitamin A (RE)*
Tomato, medium, raw (1)	75
Milk, whole (1 cup)	75
Broccoli, raw (1/2 cup)	70
Green bell pepper, raw (1/2 cup)	30
Collards, frozen, boiled (1/2 cup)	30
Orange, medium (1)	30

* The vitamin A content of food is measured in both Retinol Equivalents (RE) and International Units (IU). The Recommended Dietary Allowances (RDAs) are expressed in REs, while the % Daily Values—used on food labels and many dietary supplements—are based in IUs.

Many fortified foods, including breakfast cereals, are sources of vitamin A, too. Read the Nutrition Facts panel on food labels to see how much they supply.

Vitamin C: Not Just From Citrus!

Citrus fruit—orange, grapefruit, tangerine—are well-known sources of vitamin C, also known as ascorbic acid.

Most healthy adults age 15 and over need about 60 milligrams of vitamin C daily. Look for these fruit and vegetable sources, too.

Food	Vitamin C (mg)
Guava, medium (1)	165
Red bell pepper (1/2 cup)	95
Papaya, medium (1/2)	95
Orange juice, from frozen concentrate (3/4 cup)	75
Orange, medium (1)	60
Broccoli, boiled (1/2 cup)	60
Green bell pepper (1/2 cup)	45
Kohlrabi, boiled (1/2 cup)	45
Strawberries (1/2 cup)	45
Grapefruit, white (1/2)	40
Cantaloupe (1/2 cup)	35
Tomato juice (3/4 cup)	35
Mango, medium (1/2)	30
Tangerine, medium (1)	25
Potato, baked with skin (1)	25
Cabbage, raw (1/2 cup)	25
Tomato, medium, raw (1)	25
Collard greens, frozen, boiled (1/2 cup)	25
Spinach, raw (1 cup)	15

Some fruit drinks and other processed foods are fortified with vitamin C. Check the Nutrition Facts panel for the amount per serving. And remember, if you rely only on fortified foods as your vitamin C source, you may miss out on other nutrients and compounds present in foods with naturally occurring vitamin C.

Calcium: How Much in Food?

You need calcium for healthy bones now, as you did during childhood. How much depends on your age and stage in life. Here's the amount recommended by the National Academy of Sciences:

Age	Calcium (mg/day)
9-18	1,300
19-50	1,000
51+	1,200
pregnant and breast-feeding women (19-50)	1,000
pregnant and breast-feeding adolescents (≤18)	1,300

Dairy foods supply 75 percent of the calcium in the U.S. food supply. They also supply protein, vitamin D, and phosphorus, which together help the body absorb and deposit calcium in bones.

Other foods also supply calcium, including some deep green leafy vegetables and fish with edible bones. However, some vegetables, such as spinach, contain oxalates; grains may contain phytates. Both bind with some minerals, including calcium, magnesium, and iron, partially blocking their absorption. Many processed foods, such as orange juice and breakfast cereal, may be fortified with calcium.

Food	Calcium (mg)
Yogurt, plain, nonfat (1 cup)	450
Yogurt, plain, low-fat (1 cup)	415
Yogurt, fruit (1 cup)	315
Milk, fat-free, 2%, whole (1 cup)	290-300
Chocolate milk, 1% or 2% (1 cup)	285
Calcium-fortified soy milk (8 ounces)	250-300
Swiss cheese (1 ounce)	270
Tofu (made with calcium sulfate, 1/2 cup)	260
Calcium-fortified orange juice (3/4 cup)	225
Cheese pizza (1/8 of a 15-inch pizza)	220
Cheddar cheese (1 ounce)	205

About Some Nutrients in Food

Food	Calcium (mg)
Salmon, canned with edible bones (3 ounces.)	205
Mozzarella cheese, part skim (1 ounce)	185
Blackstrap molasses (1 tablespoon)	170
Pudding (1/2 cup)	150
Frozen yogurt (1/2 cup)	105
Turnip greens (1/2 cup)	100
Sardines with edible bones (1 ounce)	90
Ice cream (1/2 cup)	85
Dried figs (3)	80
Cottage cheese (1/2 cup)	75
Tempeh (1/2 cup)	75
Parmesan cheese (1 tablespoon)	70
Mustard greens (1/2 cup)	50
Okra (1/2 cup)	50
Orange (1)	50
Broccoli or kale (1/2 cup)	45
Anchovies with edible bones (5)	45
Tortillas (made from lime-processed corn)	40
Pinto beans (1/2 cup)	40

Iron...From Many Sources

Iron comes from foods of both plant and animal origin. Iron from meat, poultry, and fish is mostly heme iron. Usually it's better absorbed than non-heme iron from plants and egg yolks.

Many foods are enriched or fortified with iron: iron-enriched flour (also used in baked goods and pasta) and iron-fortified breakfast cereals.

Teen and adult women (up to age 50 or so) need about 15 milligrams of iron daily. During pregnancy, iron needs increase to 30 milligrams daily. Teenage boys need about 12 milligrams of iron each day. And men, as well as women from 51 on, need about 10 milligrams of iron daily.

Food	Iron (mg)
Sources of Mostly Heme Iron	
Beef liver, braised (3 ounces)	5.8
Lean sirloin, broiled (3 ounces)	2.9
Lean ground beef, broiled (3 ounces)	1.8

Food	Iron (mg)
Skinless chicken breast, roasted dark meat (3 ounces)	1.1
Skinless chicken breast, roasted white meat (3 ounces)	1.0
Pork, lean, roasted (3 ounces)	1.0
Salmon, canned with bone (3 ounces)	0.7

Sources of Non-Heme Iron

Food	Iron (mg)
Fortified breakfast cereal (1 cup)*	4.5-18
Pumpkin seeds (1 ounce)	4.3
Bran (1/2 cup)	3.5
Blackstrap molasses (1 tablespoon)	3.5
Soybean nuts (1/2 cup)	3.4
Spinach, boiled (1/2 cup)	3.2
Red kidney beans, cooked (1/2 cup)	2.6
Lima beans, cooked (1/2 cup)	2.5
Prune juice (3/4 cup)	2.3
Pretzels (1 ounce)	1.3
Enriched rice, cooked (1/2 cup)	1.2
Raisins, seedless (1/3 cup)	1.1
Prunes, dried (5)	1.1
Whole-wheat bread (1 slice)	0.9
Green beans, cooked (1/2 cup)	0.8
Egg yolk, large (1)	0.7
Peanut butter, chunky (2 tablespoons)	0.6
Apricots, dried (3)	0.6
White bread, made with enriched flour (1 slice)	0.7
Cod, broiled (3 ounces)	0.4
Zucchini, cooked (1/2 cup)	0.3
Cranberry juice (3/4 cup)	0.2
Unenriched rice, cooked (1/2 cup)	0.2
Grapes (1/3 cup)	0.1
Egg white, large (1)	< 0.1

* Amount varies. Read the Nutrition Facts panel.

Food's Fiber Factor

Many health experts recommend 20 to 35 grams of fiber daily. Yet the average American diet supplies only half that much.

Fiber comes from plant sources of food: whole-grain products, legumes, vegetables, and fruits (especially with edible peels on).

Consider these common sources of fiber:

	Amount	Fiber* (g)	Calories
Fruits			
Apple (w/skin)	1 medium	3	80
Applesauce	1/2 cup	2	55
Banana	1 medium	2	105
Blueberries	1/2 cup	2	40
Cantaloupe	1 cup	1	60
Figs, dried	2	4	95
Grapes	1/2 cup	1	30
Orange	1 medium	3	60
Orange juice	3/4 cup	< 1	75
Peach (w/skin)	1 medium	1	40
Pear (w/skin)	1 medium	4	100
Prunes, dried	3	2	60
Raisins	1/4 cup	2	115
Strawberries	1 cup	4	45
Vegetables, cooked			
Broccoli	1/2 cup	2	25
Brussels sprouts	1/2 cup	3	30
Peas	1/2 cup	2	65
Potato, baked (w/skin)	1 medium	4	200
Potato, mashed	1/2 cup	1	110
Spinach	1/2 cup	2	20
Sweet potato, baked (w/skin)	1/2 medium	2	60
Zucchini	1/2 cup	1	20
Vegetables, raw			
Carrots	1 medium	2	30
Celery	1 stalk	< 1	5
Cucumber, sliced	1/2 cup	< 1	5
Lettuce, romaine	1 cup	1	10
Mushrooms, sliced	1/2 cup	< 1	10
Spinach	1 cup	1	10
Tomato	1 medium	2	30
Legumes, cooked			
Baked beans, plain or vegetarian	1/2 cup	3	120
Kidney beans	1/2 cup	3	115
Lentils	1/2 cup	4	115

	Amount	Fiber* (g)	Calories
Breads, grains, and pasta			
Bagel	1 medium	1	165
Bread stick	1	< 1	115
Brown rice, cooked	1/2 cup	2	110
French bread	1 slice	< 1	80
Pumpernickel bread	1 slice	3	80
Spaghetti, cooked	1/2 cup	1	100
Wheat bran	1 tablespoon	2	10
Wheat germ	1 tablespoon	1	15
White bread	1 slice	< 1	60
White rice, cooked	1/2 cup	1	135
Whole-wheat bread	1 slice	2	60
Breakfast cereals			
100% bran	1/3 cup	8	70
Bran flakes	3/4 cup	5	90
Corn flakes	3/4 cup	1	100
Granola w/raisins	1/4 cup	2	130
Oatmeal, cooked	3/4 cup	3	95
Raisin bran	3/4 cup	5	120
Snack foods			
Hummus dip	2 tablespoons	2	50
Peanuts, dry-roasted	1/4 cup	3	215
Popcorn, air-popped	1 cup	1	30
Sunflower seeds	1/4 cup	2	210
Walnuts	1/4 cup	1	95

*Due to the different methods used in determining fiber in foods, fiber values found on Nutrition Facts panels and in other sources of fiber information may vary slightly from those listed.

Note: Nutrient values are rounded.

Sources: *Bowes & Church's Food Values of Portions Commonly Used, 16th Edition*, 1994; *Plant Fiber in Foods*, 2nd Edition, 1990; and manufacturer data.

Sodium: In Which Foods?

We need sodium to be healthy. Yet, most Americans consume far more than they need. Because high blood pressure is linked to eating too much sodium among some people, health experts advise just moderate amounts: 2,400 milligrams or less a day.

While fresh foods are lowest in sodium, processed and prepared foods can be part of your healthful eating plan, too. But some processed foods have more sodium than others: including cured and processed meats; canned foods, such as legumes, vegetables, and fish; cheese; condiments; convenience foods, such as pasta mixes or rice side dishes; and salted snack foods. Note these differences in similar products.

Food	Sodium (mg)
2 ounces canned tuna	310
2 ounces low-sodium canned tuna	135
1 medium dill pickle	835
1 medium cucumber, marinated in vinegar	5
3 ounces ham	1,030
3 ounces lean pork loin	75
3 cups regular microwave popcorn	190
3 cups air-popped popcorn	< 5
3 cups salt-free microwave popcorn	0
1 cup boxed convenience rice	1,600
1 cup plain brown or white rice	5
1/2 cup canned green beans	170
1/2 cup frozen green beans	5
1/2 cup fresh green beans	<5
1/2 cup canned no-salt-added green beans	<5
1 cup chicken broth	1,005
1 cup low-sodium chicken broth	70

When You Need to Know More

Healthy Weight
—For You!

THERE'S NO SPECIFIC WEIGHT that's right for your age, sex, and height. And there's no single reason why weight differs from person to person. Your healthy weight depends on several factors, including where your body fat is located, how much of your weight is fat, and if you have weight-related health problems, such as diabetes or high blood pressure. To help you judge your current weight:

➤ Give yourself a mirror test. Are you shaped like an apple or a pear? Extra body fat around the midriff is riskier than extra fat around the hips, buttocks, and thighs. Measuring your waist-to-hip ratio is another way to tell. Refer to page 6.

➤ Compare your weight with a weight chart. Refer to page 6 in "All About You."

➤ Talk to your physician about a healthy weight for you and your overall health.

Seven Questions to Ask About
Healthy Weight Management

Whether you need to lose, gain, or maintain your healthy weight, manage your weight safely and effectively for the long term. You should be able to answer "yes" to the following seven questions. Does your plan...

➤ Include a variety of foods from all five food groups of the Food Guide Pyramid?

➤ Offer appealing foods to enjoy for the rest of your life, not just for a few weeks or months?

Just Having Food Around. If the sight of chips, candy, and other high-calorie foods lures you, even when you're not hungry, keep them in an inconvenient place. Remember, out of sight, out of mind!

Mindless Nibbling. Like to nibble while you read, do paperwork, or watch TV? Instead of snack beverages or foods, keep a glass of water handy.

'Tis the Season. Watch for seasonal triggers: a six-pack of beer during hot weather, or snacking as you watch winter sports, or holiday celebrations.

When You Need to Know More

How to Get Sound Advice About Healthful Eating

KEEPING A DAILY FOOD AND PHYSICAL ACTIVITY RECORD may prompt questions about eating for health, or perhaps your desire for advice from a qualified nutrition expert.

Qualified nutrition experts have academic training and credentials in nutrition, dietetics, or related fields, such as public health, biochemistry or a nutrition specialty in family and consumer sciences. Their degrees come from accredited colleges and universities. Among those qualified to offer nutrition advice are registered dietitians (RD) and dietetic technicians, registered (DTR).

To find reliable answers and sound, scientifically-based nutrition guidance, contact:

➤ your doctor, health maintenance organization (HMO), or local hospital for a referral

➤ your local dietetic association, public health department, extension service, or the nutrition department of an area college or university

➤ The American Dietetic Association/ National Center for Nutrition and Dietetics. Ask for a referral to a registered dietitian (RD) in your area.
   —Consumer Nutrition Hot Line at 800/366-1655
   —On-line: http://www.eatright.org

Index

activity assessment, 7–8
activity goals, personal, 8
activity strategies, 34–35
activity, 29–32
  benefits of, 29–30
  everyday tips, 49, 53, 57, 61, 65, 69,
    87, 91, 99, 109, 117, 121, 129,
    143, 147, 159, 173
  moderate (table), 31
alcoholic beverages, 27
American Dietetic Association, v, 199
assessments,
  activity, 7–8
  nutrition, 3–6
  weight, 6

beans, 22–24
beta carotene, 19, 20, 59,
  187–188 (table)
beverages, 27–28
bicycling tips, 103
Bread Group, 18–19, 184
breakfast, 63

caffeinated beverages, 27
calcium, 21, 119, 180–190 (table)
  recommendations, 189
calorie recommendations, 14, 15–16
carbohydrates, 18, 20
cereal, 18–19

cheese, 21–22
cholesterol, dietary, 183–187 (table)
combination foods, 24–25
cooking tips, low-fat, 97, 123

dance, 69, 109
Dietary Guidelines for Americans, 11
dieting, 105
dining out tips, 55, 145, 149

eggs, 22–24
ethnic foods, 175
exercise strategies, 34–35
exercise videos, 83
exercise, 29–32 (see also activity)
  benefits of, 29–30

fat, dietary, 71, 183–187 (table)
Fats Group, 24, 186–187
fiber, 18, 20, 191–193 (table)
  recommendations, 191
fish, 22–24
  consumption tips, 137
fitness, definition of, 1
fluids, 27–28
folic acid, 19, 20
Food Guide Pyramid, 12–28
food groups, Pyramid, 13–14, 16–24
Fruit Group, 20–21, 185
fruits, consumption tips, 51, 89, 101,
  141

gifts, food-related, 171
goals, personal nutrition and activity, 8, 15–17, 35–38, 75, 105, 135, 165, 179
grains, 18–19, 107
    consumption tips, 153

housework activity and, 57

iron, 18, 22, 190–191 (table)
    recommendations, 190

legumes, 22–24, 107
lunch tips, 89

Meat Group, 22–24, 185–186
meat consumption tips, 157
meat rubs, 67
Milk Group, 21–22, 185
milk, consumption tips, 131
muscle, 135

nutrients, 183–194 (tables)
nutrition advice, seeking, 199
nutrition assessment, 3–6
nutrition goals, personal, 8
nutrition strategies, 33–34, 197–198
nuts, 22–24

oils, cooking, 24

pasta, 18–19
portions,
    Bread Group, 18
    estimating, 26
    Fruit Group, 21
    Meat Group, 23
    Milk Group, 22

tips, 115, 149, 165
    Vegetable Group, 19–20
potassium, 20
poultry, 22–24
    cooking tips, 81
pregnancy, 14, 19

record keeping strategies, 39–41
rice, 18–19
rubs, meat, 67

salad tips, 93
servings recommendations, food, 14–17
shopping tips, food, 55
snack tips, 85, 89, 101, 161
sodium, 193–194 (table)
    recommendations, 193
sweets, 24

tofu, 22–24
travel tips, 65, 95, 155, 177

Vegetable Group, 19–20, 184–185
vegetables
    consumption tips, 47, 51, 59, 101
vitamin A, 19, 20, 59, 187–188 (table)
vitamin B, 18
vitamin C, 19, 20, 188–189 (table)

waist-to-hip ratio, 6–7
walking, 53, 79, 125, 133, 151, 163, 169
weight assessment, 6
weight management, 195–196

yogurt, 21–22

zinc, 22–23

More Nutrition Books
from Wiley and
The American Dietetic Association